AF352140

# THE SECRETS OF
# SUPERSTITIONS

*Other books by Owen S. Rachleff*

SKY DIAMONDS: THE NEW ASTROLOGY
THE OCCULT CONCEIT
AN ILLUSTRATED TREASURY OF BIBLE STORIES
YOUNG ISRAEL: A HISTORY OF THE MODERN NATION
REMBRANDT'S LIFE OF CHRIST

# THE SECRETS OF SUPERSTITIONS

## How They Help, How They Hurt

by Owen S. Rachleff

DOUBLEDAY & COMPANY, INC.
GARDEN CITY, NEW YORK
1976

ISBN: 0-385-11061-8
Library of Congress Catalog Card Number 75–21243

# Contents

Edgar Cayce; Occultism in Action; The Psychological Factor; Parapsychology versus Mysticism; Public Airings; Letter from a Would-be Seer.

# *Introduction*

## *Superstition—Pro and Con*

The sensible Sir Francis Bacon, in the seventeenth century, remarked that "there is a superstition in avoiding superstitions."[1] Amen. Only a kill-joy would wish to impose any stricture or inhibition on those occasional or indifferent superstitions which may be, at bottom, benevolent actions or positive rituals of deference to "higher forces" or the vagaries of luck. Knocking on wood, evading ladders, tossing salt, and "God-blessing" those who sneeze might very well fall into such a category. Casual bouts with astrology, palmistry, or the Ouija board and appreciation of the historical and artistic side of witchcraft, Satanism, and spooks may also have certain redeeming values when lightly pursued as divertissements. For its part, the "lucky" four-leafed clover, which a patient tucks under his pillow on the evening prior to an operation, may help to instill in him, unconsciously, a sense of confidence and optimism that is measurably beneficial as far as sickness goes. And if one's private little bedtime rituals aid in sleep, then more power to them. The totally antisuperstitious individual who walks about his bedroom with an open umbrella is as much a compulsive neurotic, enslaved to rituals and formulas, as the man who so fears witches and their power that he will never attend a puppet-show performance of *Hansel and Gretel.*

Extremes are extremes and should be avoided in any aspect of mental activity: superstitiousness among them. Besides, many an old wife's tale and folkloric belief comprise an art form in themselves and enrich the valuable human repository of myth, religion, and fanciful imaginings. Think where anthropology and ethnology would be without such lore. No one really proposes tampering with these qualitative aspects of superstitious conceits as they apply to human history and culture, to national aspiration, or to the age-old instinct to spin yarns and concoct tales of explanation and guidance, especially for the pleasure of the young.

However—after several years of teaching and lecturing on various phases of religion and the occult, I am inclined to recall another sensible Englishman, Mr. Edmund Burke, who warned that superstition can become, what he called, "the religion of feeble minds."[2] Intensive superstitious thinking may indeed be indicative of mental imbalance and can, even in relatively moderate cases, abet an irrational attitude toward life so that the individual eventually becomes stymied, dysfunctional, and inert—the frightened soul, for example, who perhaps unwillingly is unable to move from his bed on Friday the thirteenth in dread of the supposed disasters connected with that date. Such an extremist attitude—and it is not that uncommon, as we shall see—parallels Freud's concern about the "gap between the paranoiac's displacement and that of superstition"; a gap that he perceived to be "narrower than appears at first sight."[3]

Much narrower, I think, and in the following pages I hope to explore the nature of this diminishing gap between superstition and psychoneurosis, as well as that other level of superstitionism, the one that may be useful in coping with everyday anxieties. Accordingly, I have labeled seven superstitious types: Appeasers, Dualists, Trinketeers, Conjurors, Expiators, Stargazers, and Seers, in order to specify well-known superstitious beliefs in tandem with certain common aspects of psychology. In some cases these categories of type overlap or evolve or pass from one form to another. The Appeaser, ever fearful of natural enigma, hovers close to the Expiator's anxieties about death; the Stargazer, with his fixation on celestial fate, eventually may see himself as a Seer or prognosticator; and the uncertainties born of the Dualist view can easily pass from an obsession about Satan to the Conjuror's concerns with witchcraft and sorcery.

The psychology of superstition, however, is not only of clinical or personal interest. It has in recent times assumed wide social proportions, as witness the panic provoked by the horror film *The Exorcist,* which played on Dualist fears. Newspaper and television stories about possession, ritual murder, swindles pegged to astrology, to UFOs, hallucinogenic cults, and the fact that over a quarter million dollars of business is lost in America each and every Friday the thirteenth (because superstitious people stay at home) appear increasingly in our lives. This decidedly "medieval" temper is surrounded by a growing fascination and belief in the blandishments of witches, prophets, spirits, mind readers, key benders, stargazers, and seers. Why? What does it all mean and imply? One thing is for certain: Most of us are far more superstitious than we may imagine or ever admit, and this is not so much the result of magic or ignorance as it is a condition of human psychology on a universal scope.

## The Case of the Earth-bound Professor

A perfectly sober professor of medieval history, a friend of mine, for years avoided visiting Europe because of acute anxieties about long-distance air travel. Finally, in deference to a book he was writing on monasticism in France, the earth-bound scholar nervously and unhappily booked a seat on a 747 to Paris. The night before his departure a few of us, hoping to dispel, with wine, his preflight jitters, tendered him a private supper party.

The evening was a pleasant one so long as the conversation veered from the subject of trans-Atlantic travel, and our professor seemed comfortably resigned as he toyed with the crystal wine goblet before him.

"Well, I'd better start home and get some sleep," he finally said, "tomorrow's going to be a trying day."

Even as he spoke the word "trying" (a euphemism to be sure), the diffident pedagogue somehow managed to topple his goblet and it promptly snapped off at the stem. There was a moment of silence.

"My God," he muttered. "It's a bad omen, I'm sure of it!" Rising from his seat, pale and shaken, he asked me, as the resident expert on the occult: "Do you believe in omens?" And then, without even waiting for an answer, this sober academician, drawing upon an obviously deep-seated, perhaps unconscious, superstitious faculty, declared his intentions of canceling the Paris flight.

Now, I don't like to see a grown man, especially a learned Ph.D., capsized by superstition (my concern for the subject, as a matter of fact, is the impetus for this book), so I quickly said, "You know, of course, that the ancients very often sacrificed animals or precious objects to the gods to ensure safe travel. It was their belief that the destruction meted out upon the sacrifice would replace any disaster intended for them."

I went on to remind my friend, who was Jewish, that many a Jewish housewife, upon dropping a dish or incurring a simple household accident, will intone the protective Yiddish utterance: "*Soll sein kapporah*" ("Let that be for atonement [or future troubles]"). In short, I managed to convince the shaken medievalist that his accident with the crystal goblet could, in fact, superstitiously speaking, be a very useful propitiation against any potential dangers of his flight.

"I do remember that in Jewish weddings the bridegroom crushes a wine goblet underfoot," the professor declared, relief creeping into his voice. "I suppose that's also some sort of . . ." He broke off, searching for the correct expression.

". . . sympathetic magic," I finished for him.

"Precisely! An attempt to rearrange fate by substitutes." Then he dutifully added, "Of course, it's all nonsense," and after making profuse apologies for the broken crystal, he cheerfully went on his way —destination Paris—subconsciously assured that he had inadvertently or otherwise propitiated the antagonistic forces that lay ahead.

Naturally, one could only assume the professor's state of mind (conscious or subconscious) at that point in terms of analyzing the psychological secrets of superstitions. But assumption soon became fact. Six weeks later, the well-traveled professor safely returned to America somewhat upset because a beautiful crystal goblet he had purchased in France to replace the earlier "sacrifice," had itself been broken by him in the shop after he had paid its price.

Clearly, the myth about breaking or sacrificing a precious object as propitiation had deeply embedded itself in the professor's psychological make-up. He subconsciously reasoned, if breaking a valuable crystal goblet on the eve of his departure could effectively forestall ominous forces, then it stood to "reason" that a similar ritual, performed with the same kind of object prior to the return flight (in fact, the day before), would probably guarantee a safe landing as well. One could hardly convince the scholar that this, in fact, had been the motivation of his second accident. "Coincidence," he protested, "nothing more."

Though it is true that coincidence is a rather common fact of life, the circumstances evident in this particular example, considering the acute anxieties involved, much more favor an unconscious submission to the considerable blandishments of outright superstition.

## Standing Beyond

Before plunging into the often fascinating (sometimes frightening) world of talismans, demons, sun signs, witches, and evil eyes, we should first delineate by definition what we mean by superstition and how this word may be scientifically applied. In doing so, we will inevitably skirt the borders of religious and cultural beliefs. We are well advised to do so, since these borders are often booby trapped with irrational (and therefore dangerous) ingredients; articles of faith that soon become superstitions, that prey on the mind and actually inhibit by anxiety a mature and productive existence. Such areas are, of course, highly controversial. When is something merely a superstition and when is it a cherished religious or cultural ideal? As far back as the seventeenth century Thomas Hobbes made a useful distinction. Writing in his *Leviathan*, he said: "Fear of power invisible, feigned by the mind or imagined from tales publicly allowed, [is] religion; not allowed, superstition."[4]

Hobbes's parallelism gets us to the etymology of the word itself. Superstition, from the Latin *super-stit,* simply means "standing beyond," or above, in the sense of beyond the normally enlightened values of a given time or place. The word "heathen" (*paganus* in Latin) neatly relates to *super-stit* since heathens were considered outcasts and oddballs, who practiced their weird beliefs "up on the heaths," out of the sensible community locus. In the Middle Ages, when the Church established an order of demonologists, who in turn established an order of demons, Beelzebub, the beneficent "Lord of the Flies" of Canaanitish worship, became the Prince of the Devils, "one next himself in power, and next in crime" to Satan, as Milton reports in *Paradise Lost.* So it may follow that astrology in one period, let us say around 900 A.D., is regarded as a science in Europe, while the worship of the Egyptian sun god Ra at the same time is condemned as a loathsome superstition. The principle that seemingly prevailed in the past regarding the distinctions between superstitions, religions, and scientific fact had to do with credibility and acceptability—or to use Hobbes's neat phraseology—what was publicly allowed as opposed to that which was taboo. This basic distinction must apply even today with one further essential consideration: scientific evidence. By such means we can show that astrology, as popularly practiced, is based on outdated astronomical information and faulty geophysical conclusions. If its practitioners insist that astrology works, then, in light of the inescapable scientific evidence mounted against it, it must work by the dubious laws of some magical or metaphysical system gradually disallowed by enlightened men and women of the twentieth century. Astrology is therefore a superstition belonging to a series of "beliefs or practices groundless in themselves and inconsistent with the degree of enlightenment reached by the community to which one belongs," to quote the Encyclopedia Britannica under "Superstition."[5] In short, for our purposes, superstition simply means a belief beyond rational understanding. It does not necessarily imply any shameful status, no matter how much a problem it may be.

## Of Blessings and Curses

To cope with the variety of superstitious experiences, past and present, this book will be divided into chapters that embrace each of the general categories of belief patterns that play a viable role in human psychology: superstitions derived from religion (both pagan and the Judeo-Christian variety); those of more cultural origins and effects; those linked to witchcraft and the sexual instinct; superstitions of cosmic proportions, including astrology, numerology; and those that deal with death and the afterlife—death being one of the fundamental wellsprings of all superstitious consideration—as well as the more popular notions about mirrors, names, charms, and air travel.

These categories will not consist of mere listings in the style of a Gilbert and Sullivan patter song (I'm thinking of John Wellington Wells, the sorcerer, and his long catalogue of magical nostrums). They will hopefully represent discernible elements in a blueprint of personality, including specification of different superstitious types, the aforementioned Appeaser, Expiator, Trinketeer, and so forth. By understanding the psychological common denominator of superstition and of these types, one can evaluate one's own personality inclinations as regards the general phenomena of "credology"—which is my own word for *what people believe.* In addition, by accepting the explanation of their sources, motivations, accretions, and their delusory problems in general, one can, hopefully, overcome faulty superstitious influence, real or potential, and remove yet another incipient virus from the realm of mental health.

Mental health is the goal of this endeavor, and I do not think it either a presumptuous or overly dramatized goal. As I have said, in my dealings with persons concerned and deeply involved with both religion and the occult, I have found an alarmingly high proportion veering toward symptomatic affects of mental disturbance. In my studies with psychotherapists, I have seen a parallel incidence of eccentric religious and superstitious beliefs among persons professionally diagnosed as mentally ill. Psychoanalysts believe some form of sexual maladjustment to be concomitant with psychoneurosis. I venture to suggest that serious superstitious dependency is a similar concomitant factor in almost every case of personality disturbance. With such ominous possibilities at play and considering the current proliferation of occultic ideologies, any means of mitigating harmful superstitious symptoms should be as welcome to the general reader as the authoritative sex manual which helps him adjust to, debunk, or place in proper perspective the sexual side of existence.


## *The Paper Crutch*


Frequently we hear about the dangers of smashing people's illusions, leaving the individual high and dry without his fantasies or dreams in the name of rationalism and truth. Is there not, in itself, some invidious effect that may result from debunking and depropagandizing the cherished myths of credology, just as there may be compulsion attached to complete avoidance of superstition per se?

In the case of the earth-bound professor, we have already reported the short-term advantages that accrued to him regarding the broken crystal and his air-flight anxieties. So far, so good. The second time the professor "accidentally" cracked a goblet, he was demonstrating, no matter how incidentally, a potential habit pattern that could result in far worse psychic problems than travel jitters. The problems I refer to revolve around the individual's inner realization of his own subtle self-deceit. Every modern astrology devotee or Trinketeer (those who crave talismans and wear amulets or lucky colors), every witch and warlock, I Ching advocate, and Tarot practitioner knows inherently that he or she is dealing in debatable realms, to say the least. All must have heard, even tangentially, those debunkers, critics, and rationalists suspicious of their vaunted enterprises. All have been called "peculiar, kooky, weird," or some such adjective even by well-meaning friends. Indeed, it seems to be the general masochistic compulsion of the "occultnik" (as I egregiously call him) to run headlong toward the pitfalls of his delusion, purposeful in the face of rationalistic antagonism and public derision. To a large degree the same holds true, these days, for the orthodox in religion. Though they may believe devoutly in their rituals, myths, and creeds, they must recognize the wide and growing spectrum of debate that pertains to their favorite disciplines. Such recognition, no matter how grudging, often tends to rankle and to diminish even the most fervent ideals, causing a reaction neurosis of potentially dangerous dimensions.

I may paint pictures or putter in the garden or play eighteen holes of golf in order to reduce psychic tension, in order to cope and simply survive. These activities function well toward the end I am seeking because they are free of psychic tensions in and of themselves—unless, of course, I become compulsive or obsessive in the process of painting or planting or putting. Certainly no one of any respectable status could debunk, or has seriously debunked, these activities or opened them to charges of deceit. I, therefore, need not harbor secret guilts about the stupidity and anility of working in oils or planting African violets or striving to improve my fairway drive. Unfortunately for them, few of those dependent on superstition are entirely free of a still small voice within that whispers, "You are fooling yourself. You know and you have heard that all this astrology or numerology and witchcraft magic is a patent fraud . . ." Or to paraphrase Ingersoll's famous description of clergymen, "They know that we know that they *don't* know!" In this case, that they—the occultniks—don't know what they're doing or why they're doing it. Often, when I have announced to an audience a lecture "Debunking the Occult," I have seen one or two timid souls quietly exit from the auditorium fearful of what they know will be a convincing assault on their delusions.

The underlying realization of the fallacy involved in a given set of beliefs causes those beliefs to become what might be called paper crutches, likely to buckle and collapse when one, of necessity, applies too much weight to them. This is a problem that afflicts more people than psychotherapists may realize or that the victims themselves and their families care to admit.

"I know it's foolish staying in bed all day on Friday the thirteenth," admits .the Seer (he who seeks omens in everything). "Ah, but if I went to work, I would probably get hit by a car or mess up my job—or who knows what!" And so this individual tucks himself safely in bed and sleeps away the ominous day. Having successfully survived his fate, the Seer in question may be led to a process of similarly reclusive solutions based on similar anxieties. Now he might decide to stay in bed on the anniversary of his mother's death, or when Saturn is in conjunction with Mars, or when the dreaded number thirteen (Death) of the Tarot pack makes itself known in a fall of cards. Before long this individual is staying in bed five days out of every twenty. Such incapacity and dysfunctional inertia perfectly parallel the external effects of illness or accident—the very problems we presume the individual was attempting to avoid. Even his job is in jeopardy as his boss becomes more and more impatient with superstitious excuses and their resultant malingering.

To be bedridden and self-deceived in the bargain! What saving delusion obtains in such a case and how misguided we are to think that we protect ourselves by leaning on paper crutches or allowing others to do the same. Happily, such instable prosthetics can be eased away from the shaky hold and replaced by the muscle tone of reality and valid information, as happened with a student of mine at New York University who objected to a classmate's allegedly "evil eye" and asked to be dropped from the course (entitled "Witchcraft, Magic, and Astrology"). Unwilling to cater to such anxieties, I persuaded the frightened woman to do two things: first, read an essay of mine on the background of the evil eye, and when that was done, to join me and a few other students for coffee after class. Having read the paper, which she admitted had been illuminating, the lady appeared after class at a local coffee shop and found herself seated across from the baleful bearer of the evil eye.

At first she protested and attempted to leave. But I prevailed upon her sense of etiquette and persuaded her to resume her seat, which she did with an averted face. Happily, the "evil eyer" was not of the Conjuror type, who believes himself empowered by supernatural magic. He was merely a studious individual with a rather fixed stare and deep-set eye sockets. Without ever referring to the problem at hand (of which I had advised him), the dark-eyed gentleman effectively charmed our frightened lady and eventually enabled her, armed with some explanatory information, to wean herself from the destructive powers of her essentially neurotic self-deceit. She was thus able to complete the course and learn even more—I hope—about the subject of superstition.

## The Social View

While the aspect of personal psychology in relation to superstition is the intended focus of this book, more sociological tangents of superstitious and fallacious beliefs cannot be ignored. Each of us is, after all, a contributory force in the social body and our own weaknesses or strengths greatly influence the health or decay of that larger sphere. As regards absurd beliefs and a general corruption of credology in the socio-politico sense, we have today at hand some startling evidence, all of it related to problematical superstitious attitudes of individuals, particularly—but not exclusively—in the United States. In early 1974, at the height of *The Exorcist* syndrome—the outbreak of latent irrationality that needed only a lurid film to be provoked—Louis Harris, the pollster, reported that 53 per cent of the solid American citizens he had questioned stated a belief in a viable, anthropomorphic Satan, and 36 per cent affirmed their faith in the reality of demonic possession. Even before *The Exorcist* burst like a flame on the lace curtains of Christian ideology, an English writer named Trevor Ravenscroft produced a fantastic, best-selling book entitled *The Spear of Destiny,* in which we are seriously led to believe that the spear that allegedly punctured Jesus while he hung on the Cross somehow managed to survive and remained a talisman for evil throughout modern history. Its last possessor was Adolf Hitler!

This explanation of Nazism and the Holocaust of World War II

is not generally known, of course, for the reason, as Ravenscroft
writes, that:

> . . . a decision had been made on the highest political level to ex-
> plain the most atrocious crimes in the history of mankind as the
> result of mental aberration and the systematic perversion of in-
> stincts. It was thought expedient to speak in dry, psycho-analyt-
> ical terms when considering the motives for incarcerating mil-
> lions of human beings in Gas Ovens, rather than to reveal that
> such practices were an integral part of a dedicated service to evil
> powers.[6]

In short, the occultic influence of this satanic spear is all we need
ever know about Nazi motivations!

Given such a superstitious explanation, considering that Satan
was essentially and inevitably responsible for the Nazi terror and
war, one might be able to forgive Adolf Hitler his crimes and lay
them to supernatural forces beyond our ken or control. By extrapolation, it may also be said that all mental disturbance and psychiatric disease—possibly *all* disease—originates in some occultic,
supernatural sphere, beholden only to its own devices and consequently beyond the tamperings of science and technology.

Superstitious belief as a way of life, as a psychological reaction
within the conscious or subconscious mind of the individual and
the collective mind of society, is but the first inexorable step toward
such a terrible, futile world view and philosophy. Carl Gustav Jung,
who attempted a psychology of beliefs, but fell victim to the occult
in the process, believed superstition rife in spite of general education and feared a "dangerous ardor" expending itself indis-
criminately in cults and irrational public practices. Even before
World War II, Jung regarded communism, nazism, and fascism as
seductive focuses for the superstitious mind. Freud, on his part,
considered superstition to be the gateway to a general, world-wide
psychosis, the tainted hors d'oeuvres to a poisonous meal. Writers
of the past, from Virgil to Bacon to Burke, and contemporary
thinkers such as Dr. Albert Ellis have perennially warned of growing dependence on the absurd, and in their respective times, have
strenuously called for a "depropagandizing" of such views. Concurrently, there have been, and are today, those on the opposite pole,
who more and more convincingly extol the virtues of magic, the
verities of so-called occult sciences, and the effective benefits of

witchcraft, exorcism, and other far-out psychic phenomena. Tangentially, but not unexpectedly, there is currently evident a new wave of fundamentalistic religious ideology, making itself felt in almost every denomination from the Westernized Krishna cults to the Jesus Freaks to a neo-Chasidic movement among Jews. These religious experiences may be beneficial in the correct proportion, especially among the young. Unfortunately, when in the realm of superstition and intense theology, correct proportion fast gives way to obsession and disease.

It is fitting on this somber note that we begin probing the "secrets" of superstitions as related to man's psychology. Society is in enough trouble these days without assuming a Ravenscroft-type analysis of its ills, an analysis which I believe simply deepens the disease. At the same time, on a less universal plane, we should not forget my friend the professor of medieval history. After all, how many crystal goblets can the old boy break before he one day severs a vital vein?

So long as man believes absurdities,
he will commit atrocities.

VOLTAIRE

# THE SECRETS OF
# SUPERSTITIONS

# CHAPTER 1

## *Appeasing the Gods*

These days, in order to witness an "authentic" pagan ritual, dramatically performed, one may find it necessary to visit an opera house during a performance of Bellini's masterpiece *Norma*. In this opera, the druidic veneration of the oak tree is depicted in some detail prior to the singing of Norma's Act I aria *"Casta Diva"* ("Sacred Moon Goddess"). Few opera lovers observing this ritual of veneration will ever realize that it is the source of one of the most popular and enduring everyday superstitions; that of knocking on wood, or "touching" wood, as the British say.

The time is 50 B.C., the setting ancient Gaul, now France. Here, the Druids, or witch doctors of the Celts, have gathered in an outdoor temple, which is, in fact, a grove of oak trees, in order to glorify their gods. The Druids believe that chief among these deities is the world creator, Irminsul, who inhabits the oak tree, an idea conveyed to them, somewhat myopically, by the fact that his visual manifestation, lightning, is frequently seen discharging itself *from* the tree on stormy nights. It is not the oak itself that is worshiped or feared; rather, the god who resides inside, along with his ominous flash, or fiery glance.

Norma is the high priestess of the Druid sect and as such must perform a fertility ritual on the rising of the full moon, which was thought to be a goddess associated with the flashy Irminsul. Because mistletoe, with its semen-colored berries, grows in tandem with the oak, Norma and her followers believe it to be the seminal duct of their god. Cutting a few branches away with a gold sickle and in sight of the moon will magically provide them, they hope, with a healthy planting and harvest as well as with bountiful human fertility. The wounded god (or tree), however, must be quickly propitiated by those who have severed his seed line. For this purpose, a pure white bull—or in some extreme cases, a virgin lady—shall be sacrificed at the foot of the tree so that it's blood, running into the earth, can restore the traumatized divinity. (I hasten to point out that this gory sacrificial service is mercifully omitted in the opera.)

Irminsul remains in his oak tree, as do countless other wood demons given birth in prehistoric times. These tree-bound forces not only emitted lightning and thunder, as the Druids believed; they also recklessly caused whole forests to burn, ravaged crops, and often threw themselves bodily upon forest travelers in the form of falling branches. And yet, despite their formidable grandeur and sacredness, and their implicit malice, trees had to be felled from earliest times in order to provide men with shelter and fuel. One after another, the godly domiciles were hacked in twain, chopped into planks and logs, and reassembled as huts and houses. Throughout the assault, however, the gods held fast to the fallen cellulose fibers and strands and continue to hold fast to this hour. Embittered by eviction, they behold the ways of men from rafters, doorjambs, chairs and tables, ever ready to emit their maledictions as of old, especially when confronted by arrogant human boasting or self-satisfaction: "That was a good harvest we had," "How well I feel today," "Your baby looks wonderful," et cetera.

Unable to sacrifice a bull or a virgin for every assault on every tree, and yet wary that the wood deities remain in their natural homes, man developed substitute methods of appeasing the gods: a stroke to caress the sacred precinct; a tap to confirm one's recognition of enigmatic forces; finally, a knock to allay their malice and propitiate—we hope—their zeal.

## The Dawn of Sacrifice

The tree was but one of the commonplace aspects of nature to confront the earliest Homo sapiens with the ineluctable enigma of life. Storm clouds, darkening skies, rain itself confirmed his abiding fears and intensified his sense of solitude and danger. The elements became, for the most part, the visual and tactile manifestations of mystery, and eventually, mystery became God. Appeasing such mystery appeared to be a sensible tack, for man had noticed that even the darkest night gives way to light, that storms eventually abate, volcanoes spend themselves, and raging fires give way to smoke. True, much damage is done in advance of such cessation; men die, cherished objects are ruined or lost, hopes are shattered. Can it be that these losses are in themselves the means of appeasing the raging elements at hand? So it seems, so it becomes. Henceforth, into the fire human beings shall be thrown; grains will be scattered on the torrents lest they rise to flood, livestock will be bludgeoned and broken in advance of the storm—all in hopes of appeasing natural forces by prior propitiation.

To be sure, these propitiations will be selective—one bull per storm; one virgin per conflagration. Selecting the one object of sacrifice, preparing it so that the elements in question might appreciate man's propitiatory efforts—all such related activities became the functions of early priests, or shamans, and the peculiar rituals that developed around these selective acts established themselves as the archetypes of religion itself.

If fertility and self-preservation informed these superstitious rituals, so did the very dawning of day or coming of night. Each was conceived as a threat to existence. In our own time, as a result, there are superstitious tendencies (and prayers) still associated particularly with the dawn and dusk: executions at dawn in order to balance the murderous vibrations involved in capital punishment with the creative powers implicit in the rising sun; the Eastern custom of measuring the beginning of day from the first hour of dusk—as consistently done in Jewish practice—signals a euphemistic appeasement of nighttime forces, as well. "We respect you, Oh Darkness, we honor you, and call you Day in the hopes that you will spare us your unseen hostilities."

The human body, from its hair to its toes, the animals that copopulated the enigmatic globe (thought to be flat in those days, of course), food, fire, pain, and sex all functioned as reminders of man's insecurity and thus reinforced his urge to appease, propitiate, and thus, hopefully, survive. The earliest attempts at such conciliation were not religious as such. They belonged to no system other than the *ad hoc* necessities of daily life. Eventually, in the form of sacrifice, they were largely incorporated into religion as we know it: the Communion sacrifice and the Passover offering are both elaborate propitiations to the enigmatic forces of spring. Even though few of us would relate the Christian Mass or the seder of the Jewish Passover to Norma's druidic activities—or with knocking on wood—they are nevertheless essentially intertwined, born of the same anxieties (performed at the same season) and dominated by man's primitive, fundamental psychology of appeasement via sacrifice. Possibly because of such latter-day religious inculcations, or because we all remain merely primitive beings burdened with history, this appeasing, sacrificing tendency loiters and lingers heavily in the make-up of the superstitious mind. As a passing adjustment to stress, such appeasement tendencies can be useful and reviving. As a dominant reaction, however, they can become a type of psychological "Munich"—an emotional sellout fraught with paranoic propensities and self-sacrifice, along with a complete negation of activism and positive thinking. The mildly appeasing superstition causes us to knock on wood; it affords us a vague, possibly humorous sense of ritual, and this, in turn, enables us to sustain the continuum of daily life without too much "hassle." Knocking on wood in this casual sense is like saying to oneself, or to the world (or even to God): "I am happy, thus boastful. But at the same time, I am cognizant of my debts to others concerning such happiness and, therefore, I knock quickly and laughingly to acknowledge these debts. It is a form of superstitious etiquette, if you will, like tipping my hat to a lady; tipping it, you'll note, not removing it entirely, thus exposing my head to the fickle elements" (a superstitious problem in itself, as we soon shall see). "It is a mere deference, a worthy sign of humility easily recognized by society as such and so rapidly performed that it is neither awkward, ritualistic, or does it become an impediment. I knock. I pass on; my self-esteem remains, my humility is appended. There is no harm."

### Faulty Psychic Action

That is putting it mildly, as said. The wilder type of Appeaser does not merely knock on wood in such circumstances. He, like the Druids of Gaul, drags forth the pure white bulls of sacrifice for elaborate, long-term rituals that inevitably tend to reinforce, by their intensities, the very anxiety one seeks to assuage. Milton said that "peace hath her victories," but in psychological terms, superstitious appeasement of a compulsive character may have only defeat and lead now, as it did in primitive times, to rigid ritualization and immolation, to a type of endless war game between the Appeaser and the primitive forces which he deems are out to punish him, even to destroy him, not for any specific crime—although the Appeaser may eventually invent such a crime (usually originating in childhood)—not because of any justified guilt-punishment equation, but simply because we pitiful human beings have been tossed, willy-nilly, into a hostile existence, which from the first (from ancient days), opposes us, fights us, embattles our souls. Accordingly, for the Appeasers, daily life is crammed with acts of knocking on wood and their personalities dominated by an unspoken formula of pacification. "Please, I beg you, oh mighty and mysterious and invisible forces of life, spare me, leave me be. True, as a child I was disobedient to mother. Possibly that is why you threaten me, whoever you are—possibly, I don't know. I know nothing about you except what my most primitive instincts reveal. When I hear a clap of thunder, when I read about a flood or earthquake, then I know you are at work. You rumble in my body, in the walls of my room—you are everywhere! And everywhere you are hostile and hidden. How grateful I am to my pagan ancestors for providing me the means of appeasing you. Their legacy remains my only hope and I hopefully proceed, immediately, to the proper rituals . . ."

Freud regarded such tendencies as "faulty psychic action," but was willing to admit that such actions could be well motivated so long as they enabled the superstitious individual to function in a productive, compatible fashion, so long as they do not "exceed a certain measure, which is firmly established through an estimation and is designated by the expression 'within normal limits.'"[1]

Granting that there are such normal limits in all superstitious types and tendencies, but at the same time warning of the abnormal "faulty psychic action" potential in most, we may now proceed to outline those early primitive superstitions that linger on and appeal most forcefully to those whom I have called the Appeaser types among us: persons who believe they are obliged continually (or frequently, depending on the intensity of belief) to propitiate negative enigmatic forces in nature and, redundantly, even in themselves.

## The Body as Bugaboo

Throughout all time, man, despite any metaphysical or philosophical and spiritual notions to the contrary, has regarded his body as synonymous with life. Indeed, a wholesome attitude toward the body may be a mark of mental health, while progressively extracorporeal, out-of-body beliefs (in ghosts, astral projections, auras, and such) often point the way to an unnatural and neurotic denial of self. Carried to the extreme, such denial has taken barbaric forms in every age and region of the world as man has branded his body, shorn his hair, suffered tattooing, circumcision, trepanation, the excision of fingers and limbs, the gouging of eyes, in the name of superstitious appeasement and self-sacrifice. Quite literally, he has transformed his body into a field of warfare between himself and the enigmatic enemy. As a result, even subsidiary body functions have been invested with occultic and superstitious qualities: sneezing, pointing, spitting, speaking, weeping, dreaming, eating, excreting, performing sexual intercourse are all involved with appeasement practices.

## Head and Hat

The head, as already noted, has been and remains the logical nucleus of magical beliefs concerning the body. Most ancients deemed the cranium to be the seat of life, of wisdom, and of the animating spirit or soul. Thus was it liable to vindictive envy by heaven-dwelling deities. Covering the head became a form of deferent appeasement and of propitious camouflage that lingers to this day in the continual wearing of the skull cap (*yarmulke*) by both pious Jews and by the leader of the Roman Catholic church, the pope himself. Muslims likewise cover their heads when in prayer and in public, and often swear by their headdress to emphasize its sacredness and self-preserving utility. Turbans, hoods, and similar caps are universally employed, ostensibly as protection against the elements in the sense of heat, cold, wind, and rain, but superstitiously in the sense of natural vengeful deities.

Of course, many may say that the practical reason for wearing a hat foreshadows any superstitious concept and that superstition is, in fact, simply a form of subtle common sense. After all, wearing a hood in the desert has a self-evident function, they say, protecting the individual against the broiling sun. Fear of supernatural forces attacking the head, it may thus be argued, is secondary to this sensible concern and was probably conceived and perpetuated as a means of instilling a useful practice in ignorant people.

My criticism with the "common-sense" foundation for superstition—wearing head coverings, not walking under ladders, not eating pork—is that even the most ignorant individual can be persuaded to cover his head under the burning sun or avoid jostling ladders lest they fall on him without further ado. Maggot-ridden pork needs no divine prohibition to consign it to the garbage heap, nor is a superstition really required to inhibit people from smashing up costly mirrors. The reason the ancients developed superstitious, that is, out-of-the-ordinary, explanations and practices in so many areas of life was not primarily for practical reasons, but for "religious" or metaphysical concerns regarding what they believed to be the supernatural vagaries of deific forces.

It should also be pointed out at this juncture that ancient peoples were not generally dualistic by belief, assigning malignant attributes only to demonic forces and benignity to the gods. Far from it. Up until Zoroaster's innovation in the sixth century B.C.—his cleavage of power into distinctly good and evil camps—all gods everywhere possessed as much malicious enterprise as creative force. Yaweh, according to Isaiah (45:7), says: "I form the light and create darkness; I make peace and create evil." From this idea, it can be understood why even heavenly forces, peering down on man's head, might be dangerous if not deflected. It should also be noted how subtle forms of deception go hand in glove with the appeasement attitude; knocking on wood to substitute a more elaborate veneration, or covering the head with a meager cap to inhibit its enviable aura or inner glow, as though the gods were so nearsighted.

But perhaps they were, for man continues in his appeasement ploys to mingle veneration with evasion and has been known in many places to thwart his gods by delectable effigies of head and skull, such as the sugar-candy skulls created in Mexico as offerings on All Souls' Day. Masks are a direct outgrowth of the appeasement syndrome related to the head. From the markings on paleolithic cave walls to modern Mardi Gras festivals, we can see evidence of the mask in magical and ritual use. A primary function of these head-face coverings was to confuse the watchful deities as to the identity of the wearer. Shamans and witch doctors especially require such cautious disguise since they tend to tamper with mysterious domains usually reserved to enigmatic nature. Elaborate make-up, especially as worn by women (male courtiers also wore heavy face paint in Europe until the French Revolution), serves as an unconscious modern substitute for the protective mask. Two related forms of protection are implied by this idea; first, that individual wishes to defend the public orifices of his body against malignant intrusion. Thus it is that red paint, which resembles life-giving blood, on the lips wards off demons who might enter through the open mouth. Second, there is the desire to keep the gods and/or demons peaceful by pretenses of self-mutilation; streaks of blood (in reality pigment) across the lips and cheeks, on the forehead, over the eyes, even on the fingertips might take the place of actual scars and bruises, such as those inflicted during propitiatory puberty rites in many aboriginal cultures. Of course, these cosmetic ploys are indicative of human sacrifice, the ultimate—and most psychopathic— or appeasing rituals.

## Hair and Beard

Crowning the head as a sort of outgrowth of its magnificence, is the hair, a part of the body long invested with magical and thus superstitious qualities. Ancient man was quick to note, in this area, that immature boys and eunuchs possessed neither body hair nor virility, establishing hair as a "macho" symbol. Illness that caused depilation was regarded with disdain, including loss of hair by women as well as men. The psychological traumas resulting from early baldness or shorning were also taken into account in the development of hair-related phobias. Samson's fate in this regard is too well known to be repeated in detail, except to say that his own maladjustment—superstitiously motivated in part—to the famous haircut no doubt disoriented his self-confidence, ergo his strength, and left him unnecessarily at the mercy of his enemies.

Many primitive peoples believe the hair to possess aspects of the soul, and because of its intimacy with the flesh, but lack of similar sensation, hair became a noble and propitious sacrifice to the gods. The story of Queen Berenice of Egypt comes to mind. In dutiful prayer that her soldier husband might return safely from battle, Berenice snipped off her luxuriant braids and laid them on the altar of Venus. In due course, when the priests went to the temple, they learned that the braids had vanished and were nowhere to be found. When Berenice's husband returned safely, it was discovered that Venus herself, deeply touched by the extent of the sacrifice, had taken the lovely tresses to heaven and laid them out among the stars. The constellation Coma Berenices (The Braids of Berenice) still shine forth in memory of this mythical deference.

Because the hair so closely represents the body, to this day many consider it unlucky to cut the hair (especially of the face) lest it fall into the hands of enemies who may, by sympathetic magic, utilize pieces of hair in preparing malignant charms against the owner. (This is believed true of nail parings as well.) In ancient times when hair was cut, the by-products were burned to prevent misuse. For ultimate protection in this regard, simply not cutting the hair in the first place seemed the most logical course and the one that also best deferred to nature. Men reasoned that since face hair grew despite shaving, the gods apparently wished it so and would brook no artificial interference. Conversely, because nature did not encourage facial hair on women, all those unfortunate females who sported incipient mustaches and beards must perforce be evil and depraved. In the fourteenth and fifteenth centuries, such women were condemned as witches; their hairy warts and stubbled chins offered as evidence of their witchery.

Some cultures were obliged to compromise with hair taboos owing to climate and other physical conditions. The ancient Egyptians apparently disliked body hair in the heat and women as well as men preferred to be depilated from the tops of their heads to their pubic regions. However, deference to the sacredness of hair never waned even under such considerations. Elaborate wigs, false beards, eyelashes, and the like were created to salve the offended gods, whom the Egyptians believed had a special affinity for hair. Even the Egyptian queen Hatshepsut wore a false beard, as her extant statuary shows.

When one regards history through art, it becomes obvious that clean-shaven faces and closely cropped hair styles for men are the exception, rather than the rule. Modern face shaving probably began in earnest when Queen Elizabeth I decided to tax all Englishmen who sported beards. Even then, most of the great Elizabethans who come to mind (Shakespeare, Raleigh, Essex, among others) maintained their face hair to some degree.

In modern religious terms, the hair still functions as a propitiatory symbol. The Orthodox Jew considers beards and the forelocks sacred and untouchable. From infancy, he is encouraged to cultivate his *payess* (forelocks) so that they may frame his face in luxuriant curls by manhood. Orthodox Jewish women, on the other hand, were shorn at marriage, (some still are), but their own hair was then fashioned into a wig, which was thereafter worn through life. This shorning served as a form of wedding sacrifice, a propitiation like surrendering the hymen (the veil) or the dowry. Face hair is also sacred in Islam and among many black Africans. Rare it is indeed to see a mature Arab male without at least a mustache, and the same may be said of many blacks.

Appeasers unconsciously regard their hair as both protective and fortunate in nature. This may be one reason for the revival of shoulder-length hair among young males in recent times. For them, long tresses mean protected and lucky independence, especially from military service, the physical symbol of which is the crew cut (as it is of prison life). If you wish to offend God and nature, the Appeaser says, cut your hair or disfigure it. Then you join the ranks of those who mourn and who cut their tresses accordingly or those defiled by enemies, i.e., who have been scalped, or drafted or imprisoned, or perhaps enslaved to Establishment jobs that still demand the all-American clean-cut appearance. By resembling these "unfortunates," you tempt fate to convey their misfortunes to you.


### Eye for an Eye


In similar ways, other parts of the body are viewed in superstitious terms as either propitious when whole and deferent, or troublesome when altered and rebellious. The eye, as the proverbial window of the soul, is a major focus of such concern and the "evil eye," as explained in the Introduction still holds sway as a magical and neurotic symbol from its Italian version *malocchio* to the Hebrew *ayn hara*. One can imagine how our primitive ancestors related the eye to the enigmatic forces of nature, for it is the eye that often most clearly delineates the oncoming storm, the smoldering fire, the puzzling contrasts of light and darkness, of human behavior, of animal life. The smallest details of our strange and wonderful existence are first and best perceived by vision. If this is so, God's eye must then be a millionfold more perceptive than ours. He sees all, whether he is the Egyptian sun god Ra, whose eye was curative as well as omnipresent, or Brahma, the Hindu creator, "whose eye controls this world" (Rig-Veda), or Yaweh whose "eyes . . . are in every place beholding the evil and the good" (Prov. 15:3), or the Nordic Odin, who sacrificed one of his eyes in exchange for immortal wisdom. If such deific eyes see all and are at the same time potentially punishing, what better sacrifice than vision itself to propitiate the god behind the eye? A sort of "eye for an eye" philosophy develops between man and the omniscient, best exemplified in legend by Oedipus, who blinds himself to appease the furies for his sins. Externally inflicted blindness may also be associated with punishment for offending nature and the gods "face to face." Tiresias was blinded by Athena because he gazed upon her naked body as she bathed. Likewise, Leviticus in the Old Testament equates looking upon nakedness with sin and with punishment (20:17). It follows that the superstitious person comes to believe that the eye must avoid sight of forbidden objects, the nude body pre-eminently, again in deference to godly restrictions. Only the deities may look upon wondrous nature in its entirety and behold all that is under the sun and in the hearts of men. The witch and wizard, who have balefully developed their evil eyes, expropriate these tabooed functions and are thus accursed, some even blinded, as was Elymas the sorcerer in the Book of Acts (13:8–11).

The lascivious eye is likewise often blinded or goes awry. Consequently, the casual Appeaser averts his eyes, especially from other eyes, in the same way he may knock on wood. More intensely superstitious persons, fearing to look upon the face of God (a great offense in many cultures), develop a sort of superstitious blindness or blindspot to many subtle aspects of nature. They will not look upon their own nakedness in a mirror, or upon public acts of urination (even of animals), or upon love-making, their own or anybody else's, lest they become accursed voyeurs. Scrutinizing someone's eating habits may also be considered beyond the realm of the ordinary eye. One should note here how everyday etiquette, as preached by Emily Post and others, plays its part in reinforcing these taboos, denoting as "impolite" any acts of staring or peeping at natural functions and activities. This is an outgrowth of the appeasement syndrome, the fear of offending enigmatic forces by "seeing too much" in imitation of the all-seeing gods.

## Heart and Blood

If man's head is sacred because it encapsulates his spirit, his wisdom, and soul, then his heart must be of equal significance since it contains blood, the age-old synonym of life itself, "for the life of the flesh is in the blood . . ." (Lev. 17:11). From earliest times, man could equate the loss of blood with death in himself and in the animals he preyed upon. So sacred is blood in this sense that it forms a ritualistic essence in every major religion and cult activity. Christians venerate the blood of Christ in Communion (whether wine or grape juice is drunk); to the Hebrews, lamb's blood smeared on the doorposts in ancient Egypt protected against the Angel of Death (even as the blood of Christ—God's Lamb—saves from death in Christianity). Pious Jews are not permitted to taste blood in meat, for it is a delicacy reserved to God (Gen. 9:4), nor will they touch a menstruating woman in similar deference to the sacred fluid.

We have already noted the pagan reverence for blood in describing the druidic sacrifice of a bull so that its blood might renourish the oak tree. South American Indians poured blood over their altars to appease their literally bloodthirsty (destructive) deities. The blood-drinking vampire is a modern myth born of primitive religious belief that originated in Mesopotamian concepts of the undead who could not thrive without transfusions from the living. Even in Hinduism, a religion not overly concerned with such matters, blood is equated with the soul that rises like a bright red flame from the wounded body and forms a sacred entity in the karma, or reincarnation cycle.

## Circumcision

Drawing blood as an act of propitiation is best viewed as a religio-superstitious ritual, pre-eminent of which is the world-wide practice of circumcision. Snipping or cutting the prepuce is probably a substitute action for the ultimate appeasement slaughter or emasculation of the first-born son. Abraham's preparation to sacrifice Isaac, in Genesis 22, cleary demonstrates the familiarity with child sacrifice that existed even among monotheistic Jews. The motivation behind such slaughter goes back to paleolithic times when males who had achieved dominance in a clan were likely to kill off boy babies in fear of usurpation. The god Cronus in Greek mythology, after all, usurped his father, Uranus; and Zeus, in his turn, emasculated his father, Cronus, despite the latter's attempt to rid himself of all competitive male progeny.

The reasoning (if that's the word) for first-born rituals is related to the universal veneration of first things: first fruits of a harvest, first days of the year or month, first money received in business, first love, and so forth. The first son was always of special significance, as was God's only begotten son; thus his ritual sacrifice would be surely taken by the gods as the ultimate sign of devotion and obeisance. In exchange, it was hoped, they would favor the obedient family with future healthy offspring, good crops, prosperity, and long life.

Those eschewing the outright human sacrifice (either out of consideration for sentiment or population) sought a symbolic gesture that would draw blood in a significant but relatively harmless manner. Incision on the foreskin was the favored surrogate (probably devised by the Egyptians), although scarring the skin, especially of the face, a practice known as cicatrization, often functions as well. Some cultures favor excision of the tongue, earlobe, or fingers as further circumcision surrogates.

The specifically propitiatory nature of circumcision is referred to by Sir James Frazer in his description of puberty rites in northern New Guinea. Adolescents of this culture must pass muster before a symbolic monster who is intent on swallowing them before they may reach manhood. The monster is delineated by a sort of tunnel, molded in fantastic, lizardlike shape. The initiate is forced to crawl through the tunnel, i.e., the monster's maw, to the appropriate howling of congregants. While the boy is thus "swallowed," the ritual of circumcision is performed by shamans hidden within. The incision and subsequent bleeding satisfies the monster who then spews out the adolescent prize, still bleeding from the "bite" inflicted on the penis as the initiate escaped the monster's teeth.[2]

## Blood for Life

Every modern act of circumcision, despite prophylactic claims to the contrary, is an unconscious archetype ritual of appeasement; a bargaining of blood for life, of momentary pain for lifelong prosperity. Blood superstitions in general have a similar source, including the casual wearing of red garments or objects (particularly a piece of coral), which allegedly satisfies bloodthirsty deities in some magical way, as well as the more elaborate activities which actually cause blood to flow, as in the bullfight, or in the blood pacts of friendship reportedly performed today in certain Greek letter and secret societies, or in the implications of everyday remarks, such as: "I'd cut off my right arm for him," thus offering a blood sacrifice of propitiatory significance.

The current interest in vampirism, largely stimulated by horror films, bespeaks a modern superstitious equation of blood and life along with the idea that supernatural beings can be satisfied and revivified by sucking blood. Dracula, the prototype of this modern myth, does not flourish only in fiction or films. The Associated Press in October 1973, reported a case in Hamburg where a twenty-four-year-old unskilled laborer, believing himself to be the Transylvanian fiend, attacked another youth (probably during a homosexual encounter), saying: "I am the master and must now see blood." The victim, it was reported in the press, performed obeisance to his "Dracula" in a graveyard and finally escaped to the police covered in the residue of the vampire's meal. The vampire himself was advisedly taken to a psychiatric clinic.

## Hand and Fingers

Numerous other examples of body and body-related propitiation can be cited to demonstrate man's long-term struggle with the primitive belief that nature aggressively demands our continual acquiescence.

Overly superstitious (and neurotic) people look upon their hands in this regard as frequently independent offshoots of their bodies, unresponsive to general control. Idle hands, they say, are soon put to the devil's work, and the psychoanalyst Wilhelm

Steckel relates that neurotic masturbators often blame their hands, not themselves, for autoerotic abuses. The ostensibly magical power of the hand, and correspondingly that of the fingers, derives from our unconscious recognition that the functional hand was the single most significant factor in human evolution, the factor that eventually separated Homo sapiens from all other competitive animals. Because prehistoric man could work wonders with his hands (building huts, fashioning weapons, decorating caves), he soon regarded them as sacred and accordingly memorialized the open hand by placing it on a wall, then blowing wet pigment over it and leaving a negative imprint still visible today in paleolithic caves of southern France and northern Spain.

Religious men of early civilizations equated their own hands with godly limbs and believed they could perform creative and destructive magic merely by pointing the index finger or waving the hand, presumably as the gods could do and had done. Human hands may be likewise wonderful and worthy as we know from reading the Twenty-fourth Psalm, which asks: "Who shall ascend into the hill of the Lord? or who shall stand in his holy place? He that hath clean hands . . ."; *clean* hands, not ones that have dabbled in magic and sin.

If, in fact, the hand is so wondrous, it follows that it may, like the eye, become a source of propitiation when needed. In the extreme, the hand may be hacked off and offered up in sacrificial ritual (the Romans were fond of such activities), or a finger may be so excised. On the other end of the scale, the hand may be symbolically raised in oath, extended toward heaven, palm open, fingers spread, pledging the sacrifice of grains or bullocks in deference to supernatural forces. The most common act of appeasement (or call it etiquette, remembering how etiquette reinforces superstition) is the everyday act of shaking hands. The origin of this ceremony may be traced to the fact that our primitive—as well as civilized—ancestors constantly carried weapons for protection and hunting needs. As a demonstration of interpersonal appeasement, a man might throw down his club or sword and then extend his functional hand to grasp that of his neighbor, equally disarmed.

Subconscious "handshakes with God," as we might call them, are casually and harmlessly performed each day in line with appeasement superstition. Covering the mouth when yawning, after all, derives from the fear that in the process of a yawn the soul might escape the mouth (or a life-depriving demon enter it). Yawning

Hindus will snap their fingers in front of their mouths to scare malignant forces, and orthodox Christians are reported to make the sign of the cross during such lapses. Each is acting to preserve life, which is long synonymous with religious respect and deference. Folding one's hands in prayer (a "handshake" with oneself) is more clearly submissive, more closely related to the archetypical inclination to be bound in homage to a deity, for the hands thus intertwined are unable to perform or function in their own magical way. Nor can they point and thus destroy, or rival God as a creator, nor can they take up weapons or tools, thus deflecting them from obeisance, nor may they give pleasure either by caresses or by performing everyday acts of eating, drinking, or grooming.

The observing Buddhist allows the hand to become a veritable pathway to his god and a means of signaling for himself deferent attitudes, or mudras, of homage and humility. The hands locked lightly at the finger tips, palms up in cradle fashion, is an ascetic sign, one of renunciation and piety. The right hand held against the breast, palm out, thumb and little finger touching, the other fingers raised, is an attitude of blessing; the earth-touching mudra inclines the hand downward in a relaxed, almost languid, ergo submissive, position. Superstitious Buddhists may assume such mudras and other bodily positions merely for the luck or facile obeisance they purport without the greater intensity of prayer and meditation the way a Christian may cross his fingers for luck without realizing the religious symbolization (i.e., the crossed fingers equal the crucifix) of the act.

The aforementioned "handshakes" are passingly harmless, again like knocking on wood, and often help reinforce tranquillity and a sense of homage and respect without becoming ritualistic. There is one aspect of the hand, however, that is less innocuous, and though it falls under the rubric of a later chapter, *By Lines and Signs,* it should be mentioned *en passant.* I refer to the belief that the palm reveals by its lines and mounds the secrets of the individual's personality and destiny. No wonder the hand is so eminently worthy of sacrifice for purposes of placation, especially among those who are allegedly the most expert palm readers among us, namely, the gypsies. In gypsy custom, amputation of the hand serves to punish those who offend the tribal codes (and gods). The dried-out hand of the offender, affixed with a candle between its folded center fingers, thereafter becomes a powerful and fearsome charm known as "The Hand of Glory," reportedly useful in tracking down buried treasures.

The Appeaser, in an extreme condition of psychoneurosis, may also "sacrifice" his hand without resorting to specific or literal amputation. Instead, he may subconsciously cause paralysis to overtake the hand (or other limb). Psychotherapists often tell of cases where persons who feel they have committed unwarranted acts with their hands will often show up with fingers stiffened in paralysis, thus no longer able to sin against nature (in masturbation or some other sexual act), offend the gods (by blasphemous gestures or by the striking of one's fellowman), or rival heavenly powers (creatively or magically). A useless hand is a chastised hand and self-chastisement equals appeasement in many nervous minds. (Nail and knuckle biting may be aspects of this syndrome.)

## Automatic Writing

That the left hand may not know what the right hand is doing is a maxim older than the Gospel of Matthew (where the adage appears); it is probably as old as man himself. The phenomenon of "automatic writing" conclusively demonstrates how superstition can indeed produce reactions outside the subject's knowledge or control. Though most practitioners of automatic writing believe themselves possessed by the ghostly hand of someone deceased who causes them to act as spiritualistic mediums, the fact is that profound unconscious motivations, not discarnate spirits, are the forces that propel the pen or pencil in episodes of this anomaly. An early investigator of the phenomenon, Dr. Anita Mühl viewed automatic writing as "an indicator of the fundamental factors underlying the personality . . . an especially valuable instrument in the study of mental disturbances of psychogenic origin. . . ."[3]

The study of superstitious tendencies by Appeasers to offer up the body, in part or in whole, as a means of coping with the problematic forces of existence may also be especially valuable in the study of mental disturbances. This is particularly true when these unconscious acts of self- (or body) sacrifice are intense and compulsive as in the cases of those who willingly scarify their faces and limbs, make of their heads and hair unmanageable fetishes and taboos, or indulge in self-induced paralysis, even though it be in reverence to God. "If I forget thee, O Jerusalem," sings the psalmist, "let my right hand forget her cunning." A noble thought no doubt, but when spoken by the Appeaser it might lead quite literally to a stiffened, useless limb, subconsciously and figuratively sacrificed to an all-punishing God.

### Sacrificial Surrogates—the Gods

Just as circumcision developed as a surrogate for actual human sacrifice, so other substitute forms have been sought throughout time by Appeasers who do not wish to inflict pain or harm directly on their own bodies. Accordingly, the Christian fathers of the first century, anxious to win pagan followers to their fold, abandoned the immutable Hebraic law of circumcision itself on the theory that the sacrifice of Christ was henceforth sufficient for all acts of propitiatory bloodletting. Of course, the *bris*, or circumcision ceremony, in Judaism, is not only a covenant made with God; it is also a form of tatoo, a marking that distinguishes the Jew from other nations. Pagans, because of their ubiquity, had no need of such tribal distinction, and more to the point, no desire for the pain and apparent disfiguration which the practice entailed.

The worship of those who have been sacrificed as substitutes for oneself, for example, Jesus Christ, is fundamental to many religions and may be called subliminal appeasement by means of martyred gods. The Christian church provided not only Christ as the central and supreme offering in this regard, but followed him with numerous saints who died so that others might live and propagate the faith by their example. For many Appeasers, this sort of surrogate functions admirably, and the chosen saint is quite literally adopted to stand in the subject's stead, freeing him from overt acts of propitiation and self-mutilation or disorder. Carried to the extreme, as such cases often go, the Appeaser begins to identify in all ways with his martyr-deputy and may as a result suffer the particular pains and other agonies which the saint represents. The appearance of the stigmata on the hands, feet, and face of ultra-devout Catholics bespeaks a propitiatory form of symbolic self-sacrifice not far removed from purposeful scarification. The abundance of martyred and resurrected gods in ancient times attests to the universal need for the particular propitiatory aspect of superstition now under examination. Centuries before Christ, Zoroaster, the Persian mystic, developed the notion of a Saoshyant, or Savior, a deified stand-in for the prophet himself at the final hour of judgment. Attis, the Roman pre-Christ, was sacrificed (and emasculated) at the vernal equinox, but miraculously resurrected at Easter. He commanded a wide following, as had Apollo before him (and Osiris before that). The extreme Appeasers among his devotees, in the dubious desire to imitate their god, were willingly castrated. Others, less demonstrative, merely practiced celibacy as a form of imitation and reverence. (The Attis celibates are believed to be the founders of Christian celibacy through assimilation.)

Other mythic figures throughout the world serve as sacrificial surrogates, identified with spring and resurrection, but always commanding a faithful following, which performs imitation rituals to relate them to their intermediaries more closely. Frazer tells of a Russian deity called Kupalo, who is burned (sacrificed) in effigy. Adoring devotees then leap over the fire in obeisance, thus tentatively sharing the god's own painful immolation. In our own time, a sense of identity with "sacrificial" victims may be traced in the intense, often neurotic, reactions that followed the untimely deaths of two Hollywood superstars and sex symbols (i.e., demi-gods): James Dean and Marilyn Monroe. Both have become cult figures of classic proportions, creating in their followers a desire to imitate them physically, and a philosophy that favors the Appeaser's tendency to seek a form of self-sacrifice, or—in this vein—to allow the sacrifice of another, especially of a beautiful, youthful, and sympathetic figure, to serve the same end. At the time of Marilyn Monroe's death, the press reported many expressions of "it's as though I died myself" among deeply impressionable "fans." Depersonalization, possible symptoms of paranoia, and a general attitude of irresponsibility for personal actions often result from such an extremistic conceit.


## Sacrificial Surrogates—the Animals

Less glamorous, but far more ancient, is the tendency to sacrifice animals as appeasement and as substitutes for human slaughter. Animal offerings range from the elaborate temple butcherings of bullock and heifer described throughout the Old Testament (or if you prefer, the hecatombs of Greece and Rome, in which a minimum of one hundred oxen were publicly slaughtered), down to the quaint little mummies, unearthed in London, of chickens and cats buried in sixteenth-century house foundations or chimneys as submissive "offerings" to the old pagan household gods.

The function of animals in religion and superstition is a subject worthy of a separate study. Suffice it to say that since the earliest moment of his awakening, man realized how closely his destiny was related to the beasts and birds. According to the Bible, animals were created solely for the benefit of man and intended to serve him and be subdued. Modern aborigines, and likely our own cave-dwelling ancestors, look upon the beasts of the field with greater fear and respect, for to them all creatures possess souls or animating spirits that have to be propitiated if man is ever to eat or otherwise utilize the animal's carcass. The decorated Cro-Magnon caves of Lascaux, France, depict not so much the bison and cattle per se as they do the souls or spirits of such beasts, thought to have been extracted by the magic of artistic reproduction (an idea, by the way, that causes many superstitious people to eschew portrait painting and photography lest *their* souls also be educed from them in the process).

It was not too great a leap from the acknowledgment of animal souls to the deification of beasts, such as is evident in the ancient Egyptian pantheon of animal-headed gods and in the widespread veneration of boar, lion, vulture, and serpent. Cattle also received great homage as gods (Hathor, the procreative cow-goddess of Egypt, was one) and yet were necessarily butchered for meat and hides. Ancient man was faced in this case, as he was with the felling of trees, with a conflict between necessity and reverence. Many elaborate customs have developed in our superstitious attempts to propitiate the slaughtered beasts that we eat and hunt—everything from stuffing their heads as trophies (idols?) to wearing their hides and skins in ceremonies of deference (as the ancients did), to say nothing of the specific cow worship of India, the prohibitions against eating pig meat in many parts of the world, and the current "pet craze" in the West in which cats, dogs, birds, and potentially domesticable creatures are once again revered, adorned, sacrificed for and unto, and regarded as personalities with souls and, in some cases, horoscopes of their own.

A plethora of superstitious references derives from man's fascination and fear of four-legged and winged creatures: the black cat, the dove of peace, the prophetic raven, the lucky ladybug, and all those ominous bestial denizens of the Zodiac—each with its powerful astrologic influence beaming down on the unsuspecting world. A form of sympathetic magic, in which symbolism plays a role, can also be discerned in our vocabulary regarding animals. Someone may be foxy, or snaky; catty, or bitchy; leonine or elephantine—these words relate to the belief that certain beasts possess attributes that transfer to men. Aborigines believe that the eating of lion meat will endow them with the courage of the lion, or they will dress in appropriate masks and skins to acquire the qualities of the animal in question by magic. The American Indian "Bull Dance of the Mandan," as depicted by the artist George Catlin (Smithsonian Institution), is an example, close to home, of men ceremoniously dressed in animal guises attempting to placate the spirit of the slaughtered animal. Modern man, acting under something of the same conceit, may wear a rabbit's foot in the belief that the rabbit's obvious fecundity bespeaks prosperity and good fortune (though apparently not for the footless rabbit!).

Naturally, the mimicking of a beast may lead to possession of one's soul by that beast (the werewolf syndrome); indeed, the whole question of possession in demonology (to be discussed in the following chapter) derives from these early beliefs that magically instilled the qualities of an animal into a man.

As civilization and herding replaced the random fears of nomads, animals lost most of their deific character and evolved, instead, into specific sacrifices for the very gods they once represented. We may assume that the reasoning behind such a development went something like this: If these creatures were once gods, worthy to receive sacrifice and propitiation, then surely now, when the true gods have been revealed, propitiation of these gods by means of animal sacrifice is clearly warranted. Modern echos of this concept may be found in the recognition of Jesus Christ as the *Lamb of God* (derivative of the paschal lamb offered since earliest times at the vernal equinox) and the Jewish custom of redeeming the first-born son, a deference formerly acquitted by the sacrifice of turtledoves in the Temple (Jesus was so redeemed—see Luke 2:23–24) but now accomplished with a donation of cash.

Animal sacrifices in tandem with certain witchcraft practices, or at least with practices deemed to be witchcraft, continue to this day. In 1973, I was informed by New Jersey police about pigeon and cat ritual slaughterings discovered in the Watchung Reservation and the disfiguring of horses and dogs (for satanic purposes) in a town called Somers Point, New Jersey. Regrettably, a certain amount of human cruelty and sadism plays a part in these endeavors now as in the past. But the unconscious reverence for animals as means of propitiation to enigmatic forces overrides all other ideas and lurks in the shadowy realms of compulsion—whether by bullfight or by rabbit's foot—as a means through which man may be brought in greater harmony with defiant nature.

## *Shall we Sacrifice?*

Alfred Adler in his classic *Understanding Human Nature* wrote: "There are people whose first reaction is always anxiety when they are about to begin something, whether this be merely leaving their house, or parting from a companion, or getting a job, or falling in love. They are so little connected with life and with their fellow man that every change of situation is accompanied by fear."[4]

This description can well apply to extremes of the Appeaser types who live in almost continuous alarm at what they regard to be hostile, even destructive, forces in nature. These forces are not necessarily the Judeo-Christian God or devil; they are largely pagan and animistic conceits like prehistoric tree spirits, lightning and thunder deities, and countless nameless forces and enigmas, all of them immemorial and obscure. Like shadows of the pagan past, these notions flicker on the walls of the unconscious and superstitious mind whenever basic anxiety of the type Adler describes motivates the individual. Because of their atavistic source, such ideas naturally evoke an atavistic response, one almost identical to so-called pagan rites and methodology, the chief of which is ritual propitiation or the appeasement tendencies we have been discussing. As stated, these inclinations can be passive and even productive so long as they are not subservient and born of fear. Deference to the recognition that life and living are far more complex (but not hostile) than any man may realize, no matter what his intelligence, can be a healthy and encouraging attitude. Knocking on wood thus becomes an invocation of the Confucian truth, "The man who knows what he does not know is truly wise," and not a substitute for action or an evasive submission to anxiety and unresolved dilemmas. Any sensible action that leads to permanent adjustment, to coping, and self-understanding is advisable (short of hecatombs). But, unfortunately, the Appeaser's tendency is deeply bound up in true atavistic form with the notion of sacrifice, and sacrifice—both literal and figurative—functions in psychology as a substitute and an evasion, tending to deepen the very anxieties that gave it birth. Generally speaking, the deeply appeasing type suffers from a general sense of inferiority and servility. Life for such people is a constant demonstration of suffering, chance hardship, ill luck, and meaningless disappointment. Daily vicissitudes are invariably taken as defeats, whereas the enigmas of the body and the cosmos are viewed as threats and distractions. The individual laboring under such conceptions, like his primitive forbears, is generally cheerless and heavily superstitious, seeking to make amends for the simple fact that he was born in hope of quieting the primordial storms, those that are unconsciously within as well as those from beyond.

At first, the Appeaser of this sort may be stymied by the problem at hand, the storm (or puzzle) that he believes has come blindly to pursue him. Later actions become more frenzied and apparently efficient as he begins to assemble the elements of a lifelong sacrificial procedure. In doing so, he well may adopt aspects of other superstitious types soon to be discussed, especially the wearing or possessing of protective devices and the seeking for omens and signs. He soon learns, however, that appeasement as such is not achieved lightly and demands more than the wearing of crosses and stars or the reading of cloud formations. Celibate sexual regimens, punishing severities, inertia as regards productive or pleasurable activities, and specific acts of submission, including self-victimizing rituals, may dominate this disposition. In the long run, the Appeaser is left in a state of embattlement—or, better, siege—as he finds that the myriad sacrifices, the continuous Lent-like existence, avail him little or naught. An antisocial condition may then arise; the Appeaser begins to avoid personal responsibility for anything (blaming his actions on enigmatic antagonists) and thus, while fearing any action that may offend the "gods," he seeks to sacrifice aspects of his own life or those of others.


## A Case in Point

A composite case is offered here to delineate the typical Appeaser "down the street," so to speak. Edna was raised in a fairly religious manner, but one that viewed God as a punishing, all-seeing force without much mercy or love. Her normal childhood anxieties about thunder, lightning, or explosive sounds were not coddled or mollified by her parents, who were old-school people immersed in earning their wages. Unexplained body functions, such as the onset of menstruation, frightened and worried Edna, and she never fully understood even the functional purpose of sex. In short, as she approached adulthood, Edna was identical in much of her psychological development to the aborigine or prehistoric cave dweller. Unhappy love affairs and a tyrannizing husband, whose rugged personality reinforced her views of a punishing God, led her to assume that she was simply a luckless type born to be victimized by the same inexplicable forces that had threatened her childhood.

Accordingly, Edna began to develop little rituals of appeasement centering around the pleasure-pain principle. Often she "sacrificed" eating sweets or desserts, which she loved, hoping to placate animistic forces whom she presumed were offended by her ostensible happiness. In bed with her husband, she became frigid, again equating pleasure with offense and sacrifice with deference. Her rationalization (if that is the word) was always: "better to keep on the good side . . ." Of what? Of hostile nature and the hostile gods. A miscarriage became the ultimate offering. At first it seemed to suffice on the theory, "Now I have paid my way . . . appeased the gods in the truest primitive form." But before long the event became contradictory in Edna's embattled mind. The loss of the baby was viewed not so much a sacrifice on her part as a punishment by God for faulty appeasement. And so the cycle of submission was necessarily resumed.

Perhaps the most famous and tragic Appeaser of all time—and tragedy is often the Appeaser's lot—was Jephthah, the biblical leader, who, in an attempt to placate the war gods before battle, promised to sacrifice the first thing that met him at his threshold upon his safe return from war. Jephthah had counted, no doubt, on meeting his faithful dog, a worthy though modest sacrifice, but he was met instead by his only daughter. Dutiful in the extreme, considering the Hebraic prohibitions against child sacrifice, Jephthah tearfully carried out his pledge. Like many Appeasers before and since, he based his conduct in life on an apparently inevitable balance between placation and success supported by appeasement rituals. He did not merely "knock on wood"; he instead symbolically hung himself on every tree in every forest.

CHAPTER 2

## *The Bible Says So*

The deranged reaction to *The Exorcist* was not simply the product of the author or of Hollywood ingenuity. It can also be traced to numerous passages in the Holy Bible itself. Not only exorcism and its indispensable counterpart, possession, are offered as valid phenomena by the biblical scribes, but a host of other ghostly and ghastly delusions originate in scriptural lore. Superstitions concerning ghosts, blood rites, demons, transformation, levitation, séances, swamis, second sight, and astrology riddle the sacred text and thereby take on a sort of perverse and immutable holiness, for as surely as the Bible warns against soothsayers and mediums, demons and ghouls, it also concurrently implies their *real* and functional abilities. As a result, modern witch-hunters—religious extremists on the warpath against the occult—rarely resort to scientific debunking of demons, ghosts, and the like, as they should, but rather rely on Bible-thumping prohibitions which actually reinforce, in susceptible minds, the very dangers being scorned. After all, why would Exodus 22:18 instruct, "Thou shalt not suffer a witch to live," unless the biblical scribes feared the true magic potential in such creatures? And if these God-inspired men could know such fears, then witchcraft as such must surely be valid and fearsome and not just the psychoneurotic fantasies of the sick.

Regarding superstition, the combination of biblical interdiction, on the one hand, and biblical recognition, on the other, has created a peculiar psychological reaction that has its expression in the conduct of those I call Dualists, people who base their superstitious beliefs on biblical or quasi-biblical precedences of good and evil and thus combine a pious obedience and prayer with an unconscious pagan view of the world. Often these ideas are held while the individual tries to shift immediate responsibility for his own actions and beliefs to some distant, sacred source, whether that source be God *or* the devil.

## *"God's Word"*

Naturally, Dualists have many of the traits of Appeasers. They may be by nature sacrificing, fearful, and bewildered in the face of enigmatic forces. Even so, they often show far greater resistance when confronted by the enigmatic nature of existence than Appeasers because they also believe that they have God's word to fall back upon. The problem, however, that such Dualists will face is in precisely how they evaluate "God's word" and their corresponding failure to see the *ungodly* interpretations that can derive from such evaluations.

"But we are not superstitious," the Dualists say. "We are God-fearing Bible readers. Our prayers and practices are all described in the Holy Text, where you can also find the fundamental answer to all the puzzles and problems in life, namely, the eternal battle between good and evil forces [God and the devil] essential to the Judeo-Christian faith."

Oddly enough, dualism is not essential to the Jewish faith, which invests in God alone the creative and destructive, good and evil sway. There is no Satan, capital S, in Judaic theology, only a God-directed *adversary* (Hebrew for which is *shatan*) unempowered with coequal deity. Christianity, being closer to Zoroastrian philosophy, divides the world and man's existence into perennial segments of perfect good and perfect evil. Christ in this view is all perfect; he rules and manifests all that which is perfectly good. Satan, on the other hand, masters all sin, disaster, and disgrace. In the final battle, as envisioned in the Apocalypse, Christ will triumph. But until such time, the dualistic battle rages in every corner of the cosmos and most especially in every corner of man's war-torn mind and soul.

It is little wonder, given such duality, that certain Christians of the Middle Ages, discouraged and disgusted with their faith, abandoned Christ in favor of Satan, thereby laying the bases of Gnosticism and witchcraft. Their reasoning was simple and underlies all negative Dualist beliefs even today: "If Christ [God] has failed," they said, "then we must look to the next greatest power outlined in the Bible, to Satan, the fallen angel and master over evil. His power, his magic, and even his glory are specified in the New Testament. Surely he is a worthy god when all others fail. And so we shall not be dissuaded by warnings against his powers or his works. We seek instead action, reality, and surcease from our sorrows. The Bible has given us Satan, a god; henceforth Satan we worship. Would you have us be atheists?"

Such was precisely the argument of the Cathars and other Gnostics of the twelfth and thirteenth centuries, who were often burned as heretics. Such is the rationale of modern Satanists, whose chief American spokesman, Anton La Vey, puts it this way in his *Satanic Bible*: "Modern man has come a long way; he has become disenchanted with the nonsensical dogmas of past religions [i.e., Christianity] . . . Man needs ceremony and ritual, fantasy and enchantment . . . Satanism, realizing the current needs of man, fills the large grey void . . ."[1]

La Vey is not a Bible believer, but those who are, those who take the Holy Writ as sacred in every detail and who accept it as God's unalterable word, must, by and large, walk a thin line of credulity at all times in terms of dualism and its resultant problems of psychology. We will outline and discuss these problems while retaining the highest respect for the Bible as a source of lofty inspiration, piety, and law.


## The Case of Saul


First let us look at a section of the Bible that is perhaps the most indicative of the Dualist dilemma at hand, the story of the tragic Saul, first king of Israel, who appears initially in I Samuel, Chapter 9. This section of the Bible is a sort of popular handbook of a wide variety of beliefs.

The story begins when Samuel, the prophet of Israel, is told by God to select the future king of the nation. The man he chooses is unique because "from his shoulders and upward he was higher than any of the people" (9:2). Saul's height henceforth becomes a type of omen of prophecy, even as great height is considered "lucky" in certain aboriginal tribes. For his part, Saul is convinced that it is his destiny to be king when Samuel predicts three more omens that will occur when Saul returns to his father's house; "and let it be, when these signs are come unto thee, that thou do as occasion serve thee; for God is with thee" (10:7). Is it any wonder that alleged seers like Jeane Dixon and the late Edgar Cayce, both devoted Bible readers, can prophesy "signs" and omens with impunity as did Samuel and later Saul himself (and countless other biblical seers) despite the prohibitions against divination and the fact that sorcerers are lumped together with whoremongers and murderers in Revelation 21:8?

More significant in terms of *The Exorcist* syndrome of our day is the pronouncement in I Samuel 18:10 that "the evil spirit from God came upon Saul . . ." Though essentially a poetic idea and one that tends to explain the king's psychoneurotic behavior in terms compatible with his time, this one sentence—and others like it in the New Testament—have given rise to the huge misshapen body of delusions concerning demon possession that have plagued mankind and medicine for centuries. All of them are apparently sanctioned in religious minds because "the Bible said so."

Saul's demon, just mentioned, might have remained no more than a poetic nicety for schizophrenia were it not for the Macbethian denouement of the tale (I Sam. 28), which tells of the witch of Endor and her amazing machinations. Naturally, one can read this chapter in two ways; the way a logical reader would view *Macbeth* (or even *Hamlet*); to wit: a troubled man believes himself visited by a ghost and upon hearing the fatal prophecy of that ghost sets out unconsciously to fulfill his destiny and thus perishes as prophesied. All this may be assumed from an interpretation of the biblical chapter at hand. Unfortunately, Bible believers do not interpret; they take chapter and verse at face value. By doing so, they learn from their Bibles that there were indeed bona-fide wizards and those who dealt with familiar spirits in ancient Israel and that these persons were of such authority and menace that Saul himself had them outlawed from the land. Possessed as he is, however, the king, now floundering without help from the dead Samuel, undertakes a series of divinations to discover his dreaded destiny. First, he unwisely relies on the prophetic power of dreams, then on the auguries of the Urim, assumed to be a sort of priestly crystal ball or

Ouija board. The royal prophets or "precogs" are called in; all fail to help (I Sam. 28:6). The possessed man finally seeks out a witch, despite his own prohibitions, thereby indicating his faith in the efficacy of witchcraft.

Commencing with I Samuel 28:11, we are treated to a full-blown biblical séance. The woman of Endor, who is presented as a spiritualistic medium, calls upon her control, or familiar, invokes the deceased, and then causes a rather impious vision of "gods ascending out of the earth" to materialize in her lodgings. At first Saul cannot share the medium's vision and questions her about what she sees. When she reveals that "an old man cometh up and he is covered with a mantle," Saul infers that the ghost of Samuel has appeared. At this point an interpreter of the text will point out that imagination, or suggestion—possibly hallucination—is at work and not reality. So it would seem, if it were not for the following section in which Samuel per se arises and speaks directly to Saul (I Sam. 28:15–20), foretelling his death in battle on the following day.

The Bible is subtle in idea, but rarely in plot. The reader is fully expected to believe that the discarnate spirit of Samuel has appeared to Saul just as Hamlet's ghostly father appeared to him. The fact that King Saul and his sons perish as prophesied adds to the validity of the séance scene and its ghostly protagonist. Withal, the gullible reader of I Samuel has come away from his "lesson" reinforced with the following superstitious ideas generally thought to be unworthy of sober religion: first, the powers of predicting—not prophecy in the Isaiah sense, but outright future-casting. This is followed by an avowal of omens or signs, a recognition of demon possession, a reliance on dream prophecy, use of divinational devices (the Urim), familiar spirits, séances, ghosts arising from the dead, and the general efficacy of witches, for the soothsayer of Endor surely delivers the goods despite her extralegal status. An *Encyclopedia of Occult Sciences* couldn't offer more encouragement in the baseless reliance on witchcraft and sorcery than I Samuel. Indeed, I have such a book, so titled, first published in the 1930s, which makes a point of reminding us, under the rubric "Necromancy," that "the witch of Endor raised Samuel for Saul." One senses a hint of sanctimonious respect in this reference, a well-warranted appreciation of the credibility bestowed by the Bible on the "science of raising the dead."

## *The Occult Explosion*

On the other side of the spectrum, or so it would seem, are the deeply religious types who denounce Saul for his dabbling in magic, but nonetheless completely acknowledge the power of that magic, as well as the factuality of his demonic possession, on the one hand, and of basic Satanism, on the other. One of the most popular fundamentalist Christian groups in the United States today operates out of Ambassador College in California. Their chief spokesman is Garner Ted Armstrong, a personable television proselytizer who effectively denounces the occult for its dangers but *not* for its theological humbug. In a booklet produced by Ambassador College entitled *The Occult Explosion* the dualistic dilemma is pithily (and ironically) put cheek by jowl with denunciations of witches, occultists, the practice of exorcism, and similar deplored activities. Some people, says the booklet, "consider a demonic spirit world to be a mere concept held by primitive people to explain away the presence of evil in the world.

"But the Bible does reveal that there is both a real God and a real devil . . . The existence of a devil and untold millions of demonic beings will be plain to any who believes the Bible is the inspired Word of that God."[2]

In the same booklet, the witch of Endor, per se, is regarded as a deceptive, but thoroughly effective and therefore valid, sorceress who conjures up not Samuel, but a "lying demon spirit," who apparently seems to be Samuel, although the Bible does not imply any such thing. The point here is not about lying demons versus the actual Samuel, but rather the uncanny Dualist superstition represented by the Ambassador College overview.

" . . . necromancers, even today," the booklet reveals, "profess to be able to communicate with spirits of the deceased, but *in fact* they always contact a familiar demon spirit who impersonates the dead . . ." (emphasis mine).[3]

Even so cunning an apologist as C. S. Lewis is locked into the Dualist hold when he too discusses God, Satan, angels, and devils in the Christian perception. On the one hand, he declares in *The Screwtape Letters*, he does not believe in "an uncreated being" who is opposite God, i.e., Satan. On the other hand, he believes in devils, since they are simply depraved angels and he believes in angels because the idea "agrees with the plain sense of Scripture, the tradition of Christendom, and the beliefs of most men at most times."[4]

We shall of necessity return to a fuller look at Satan and at the fruits of satanic belief, possession, exorcism, and sorcery, affording, at the same time, some biographical material on Satan that it is to be hoped will reduce his scriptural potency and thus lay ruin to a vast stretch of superstitious shenanigans. First, we should examine a treasury of absurdities regarding the occult as provided by the Old Testament and New Testament either directly or indirectly and covering all manner of madness—particularly maddening since they appear alongside such lofty pronouncements as Deuteronomy 18:10–14: "There shall not be found among you any one . . . that useth divination, or an observer of times [astrologer] or an enchanter, or a witch. Or a charmer, or a consulter with familiar spirits, or a wizard, or a necromancer . . ."

Quoting C. S. Lewis again, from the last of his Screwtape monologues: "The fine flower of unholiness can grow only in the close neighborhood of the Holy. No where do we [devils] tempt so successfully as on the very steps of the altar."[5]


## On the Altar's Steps


There is a class of superstitious people which depends on omens and divinational signs for its stability, I call these people Seers. Whether their inclination augurs well or ill for them will later be seen in Chapter 7. But should they lack for "ominous" inspiration in pursuit of specific signs or methods of reading these signs, I may advise them to join forces with their Dualist friends for a tour of the Bible, where, as already shown in I Samuel, such devices and charms are freely offered. Note that the following are not elements of religious miracle, prayer, ritual, or ideology. They are specifically occultic conceits, usually of a forbidden nature and culturally of the type rampant in the ancient world and popular even today. They are the provenance of the various soothsayers, wizards, time observers, and others referred to in dozens of biblical passages, sometimes attacked in wrathful tones, sometimes in relative recognition for magical powers (Isa. 47:13 defers to astrologers) and, at other times, as in the case of the magician-seer Balaam, with grudging respect.

## Biblical Magicians

As told in Numbers 22, Balaam is alleged to be an effective "blaster," one who can curse and bless with the aplomb of a demigod. He is hired by certain local princes to curse the Children of Israel, who are camped in the desert near Moab. The Bible never doubts Balaam's ability as a wonder-worker. In fact, God himself uses the seer to prove the holiness of Israel before its enemies by causing only blessings—not curses—to flow from his mouth. Possibly old Balaam's talents had flagged by the time of his performance at Moab. He was certainly not as efficient as the wizards in pharaoh's court (Exod. 7:11), who managed for a while to compete successfully with Moses, turning rods into snakes, or as the redoubtable New Testament grand master of magic, Simon Magus, who allegedly bewitched the people of Samaria (Acts 8:9 ff.), but who converted to Christianity in the hopes of practicing his sorcery in the name of the Holy Ghost. There is some doubt that Simon Magus was deemed a *real* wizard even by the apostles. But the damsel of Philippi, encountered by Paul (Acts 16:16), is taken for a true diviner "possessed with a spirit of divination," who manages, according to the Bible, to ply her trade effectively until exorcized.

## Patriarchs and Matriarchs

Magicians aside, there are several biblical patriarchs and matriarchs who practice divination and clearly believe in the valid working aspects of the occult. (And if they do, why shouldn't we?)

Rachel, the wife of Jacob, so deeply venerates the tutelary powers of the lares or household idols of her father that she is bestirred to steal them from his house before leaving home (Gen. 31:19), hiding them in her saddle to ensure their safety. Rachel's superstitious nature and her desperation to have a child further cause her to bargain for the supposedly magical mandrake root that her sister Leah has obtained (Gen. 30:14–16). Mandrake roots, because of their humanoid shape and allegedly aphrodisiac powers, were considered fertility charms either when worn or taken in small doses with wine. Rachel's son, Joseph, apparently born with the mandrake's aid, goes on to become something of a seer not only as regards dream interpretation, which he acknowledges to be a sacred (not occultic) gift, but in the use of a divining cup (Gen. 44: 5), a device which apparently functions like a crystal ball. The prophet Hosea implies the use of a divining staff (Hos. 4:12) and Ezekiel, who seems predisposed to magical symbolism, comments uncritically (Ezek. 21:21) on the Babylonian practices of future casting by assorted means, including the reading of animal entrails (specifically a liver).

The kings of Israel and Judah are no less inclined to the occult. Ahaziah, the son of Ahab, employs oracle readers (II Kings 1:2–6), Manasseh (II Kings 21:6) "used enchantments and dealt with familiar spirits and wizards," and great Solomon, the embodiment of sacred sagacity, seemed to have been tinged with the hocus-pocus activities of his heathen wives (I Kings 11:7–8).

In the history of magic, few characters are so admired as Solomon, who was deemed to be the founder of kabala and a magician second to none. Occultists say he cavorted with a familiar spirit called Belial and employed his own signet ring (the Shield of David), or six-pointed star, as a magical talisman. It is little wonder that many of the *grimoires*, or conjuring books, of the Middle Ages, bore Solomon's name. *The Key of Solomon, The Triad of Solomon,* are all conceived in homage to the implicit sorceries of even so sacred a king.


## *"Gesundheit"*


The Bible creates superstition apart from the specific references just cited, a problem perhaps the fault of Dualist (and other superstitious) tendencies more than of the Bible's own instruction. And yet given the deference to occult matters so far described, can we really wonder at this ironic development. Happily, most of these secondary superstitions are charming and harmless, derived more from earnest misinterpretation than from a desire to dabble in malicious sorcery. They may be called, in fact, the Dualist's version of "knocking on wood."

The practice of saying "God bless you," or some such nicety, upon hearing someone sneeze may be called the Dualist's contribution to everyday cant and it is an idea that essentially developed from a phrase in Genesis describing Adam's birth (2:7), "and [God] breathed into his nostrils the breath of life." Clearly, because the breath of life went in through the nose, then a violent sneeze might very well dislodge it. If this should happen, reasoned the sages of old, it was best to forestall damnation by a blessing for the departing soul. The Jewish flavor of this superstition is reinforced by the common use of a euphemism in place of the blessing. Pious Jews did not wish to speak God's name unless under sacred conditions. Hearing a neighbor or a kinsman sneezing was not always deemed of such moment. Instead, therefore, of "God bless you," a simple Yiddish *"Gesundheit"* (i.e., health) served as well.

## Numbering

More in tune with Dualist anxieties about satanic forces is the curious avoidance among superstitious folk of numbering or counting, or specifying anything bountiful. Both Jewish and Chinese people seem to favor this superstition; the former derive it from the biblical account of King David (I Chron. 21:1–8) and the counting of Israel. By counting or numbering his population—as a census taker does today—David apparently affronted the Lord's ancient pledge to increase the seed of Abraham. It was as though the king doubted this promise and was checking up on God. As a result, many in Israel died, probably of some plague. Consequently, pious people and others will demur if asked how many children they have, how much money they make, or how many servants, houses, friends—you name it—they possess. This cautious behavior may even extend to ordering a meal and the story goes that a certain superstitious individual, who regularly frequented a popular Jewish restaurant in New York City, habitually ordered his dinner in the following manner: "First, I won't have the chicken soup; then cancel the chopped liver; I don't want the pot roast, forget the fried potatoes with onions, omit coffee, also scratch the spongecake with honey." Fortunately, the waiter in this restaurant, long accustomed to idiosyncracies, dutifully brought forth each dish mentioned to the customer's silent delight. Chinese patriarchs, in the same manner, reportedly count their children by tapping each head and saying, "Not one, not two, not three . . ." et cetera, as David presumably should have done in I Chronicles.


## Friday the Thirteenth

The superstitious diner referred to above may have taken his "not" meal on a Friday evening to feast the onset of the Hebrew Sabbath. For most Jews this is a joyous and pious occasion. But in general Fridays have a luckless reputation, and this stems no doubt from the Sabbath observance as such. Since God rested on the seventh day after Creation, it followed that the least important day must be the sixth—the last of the great Creation week and the one, appropriately, in which man was made (Friday in Old Testament reckoning). Hebrew days begin at twilight, so that the Sabbath segment of Friday evening is distinguished from the earlier part of the day. Thus, even Jews may regard Friday, until sundown, as unlucky. Certainly Christians do, and this is because of the biblical tradition that Jesus was crucified and died on a Friday afternoon. When Friday is the thirteenth day of the month, the malignant air is multiplied by the medieval association of the number thirteen with the Tarot card of Death, which is so numbered. Also, the Last Supper, which took place in the early hours of Friday morning, witnessed thirteen at the table, including Christ. The traitor, Judas Iscariot, is usually called the thirteenth man, tying the death of Jesus to the day and to the number in an ominous and forbidding way. (This is also the origin of avoiding thirteen guests at the dinner table.)


## Scapegoats and Vipers

The seeds of superstition that flourish in the Bible—or, more precisely, in the minds of many, Bible readers—have led to bizarre activities and several of dangerous and even criminal proportions. The service of a scapegoat originates in Leviticus 16 when the high priest Aaron lays the sins of the people on an unblemished goat and allows it to "escape into the wilderness." Apparently, some sort of residual pagan practice related to a Canaanitish goat god called Azazel was memorialized by this ritual, but it came to imply, in later generations, that the sins of many could be devolved on a single symbolic victim who would then be driven away from the community. Ironically, the Jews have suffered scapegoat status more than any other people, probably because the Bible (largely written by Jews) gives unwitting credence to such a dubious practice even as it does to the intolerable notion that black men shall be slaves because Ham, whose name translates as *black,* was cursed by his father Noah (Gen. 9:22–25) to be "a servant of servants . . . unto his brethren."

Many suicidal religious cults have developed in deference to Dualist superstition, born of biblical fantasy. The most unbelievable of these groups flourishes today in the southern United States and revolves around the fondling of vipers in homage to the Gospel of Mark (16:18), where Christ tells his disciples, among other things, that they "shall take up serpents, and if they drink any deadly thing, it shall not hurt them . . . ." Somehow this phrase has come to imply that the faithful may handle poisonous snakes with impunity, and so they do, but not always without incident. Many of the latter-day "disciples" of the South are bitten by their pets, some die, though obviously these are seen as unworthy. Others live to inculcate in their children these benighted pagan practices (the Celts had a similar cult), all because "the Bible says so."

A hideous variant of this suicidal tendency related to divine instruction was reported in 1974 by the United Press International. The personnel at St. Charles Hospital, London, were shocked when a young man appeared at the clinic demanding that his arm be amputated because he had received a "message from God" so ordering. Naturally, the man was turned away. A few hours later, however, he returned with a tourniquet on the bleeding stump of his arm, radiant because he had fulfilled God's message by holding his arm on a railroad track until an unsuspecting train ran over it.

Certain persons, reacting with understandable disgust to this piece of news, might say that it was not God, but rather Satan who directed the young man in London to sever his arm, although the Bible is heavy with instances where, in fact, God himself is said to be the author of certain outrageous demands; the sacrifice of Isaac is one example. The recognition of Satan's powers in this regard, as already cited, forms the essence of the Dualist's dilemma and is the main aspect of his superstitious attitude. It deserves our special attention.

## The Devil Made Me Do It

It is ironical, if not sad, that Christianity, which presented the world with one of its most specified and exalted visions of God, should have also created a concomitant concern about Satan unparalleled in any other religion with the possible exception of Zoroastrianism, the source of dualism, and certain antique Roman Dionysian cults. The Dualist problem in Christianity was not ignored by Church Fathers who early on warned their followers that love of God, not fear of Satan, was the true path to salvation in Christ. But the continual pounding of the devil's drum, the numerous references to devil and devils in the New Testament, and the mythic fascination of the fiend, placed him in the forefront of medieval imagination despite the warnings. At the same time, satanic ideas stimulated endemic pagan ideologies of the early European Christians and generally helped to answer much about the enigma of life, no matter how negative the answers might be. Accordingly, the Dualist dilemma became an inevitable and perennial aspect of the Christian conceit.

To this day, the Manichaean battle rages particularly in relation to the superstitious psychology of our times—more and more in evidence and increasingly invested with fantasies of possession, demons, and general satanic lore. Since Satan is the ultimate focus of these attitudes, it might be advisable to trace his development briefly and at the same time, hopefully, lay to rest his assumed *reality*.

## The "Birth" of Satan

Zoroaster, born in Persia around 660 B.C., was the first philosopher to articulate a systematic view of life as a battlefield of good and evil. Identifying these forces with light and dark, he created Ormazd, the luminous god of perfection, honor, peace, and all beneficent activities, and opposing him, as adversary, Ahriman, the shadowy despoiler and negative force. When Ormazd created a rose, Ahriman burdened it with thorns—or so Zoroaster believed after a tormented youth wrestling, quite literally, with what he described as a Demon of Lies. It was this demon that the Persian mystic later, in a stroke of original but regressive creativity, renamed Ahriman, a creature coequal with God, though ultimately doomed to fail in his struggle for worldy dominance. (The Persian monk Mani, who gave us Manichaeanism centuries later, decided that the victor in the battle between good and evil was not a foregone conclusion; thus, man's destiny was ever in doubt.)

Zoroaster's black-and-white ideology eventually caught hold in Persia and was available to the Jews who were then captives of the Persian kings. Being essentially antidualist and believing the creation of both the rose and the thorn to be the province of Yaweh, the Jews rejected the concept of Ahriman, but accepted the word "adversary" (in Hebrew, *shatan*). This word, in its most juridical sense, entered the Old Testament, particularly in the story of Job. Early Christian theology had invested in Jesus of Nazareth both the nature of God and the mastery of all perfection. He was, to them, Ormazd, and as such could not be responsible for evil and corruption. Therefore, it became necessary for Ahriman to reappear as he does quite literally in Luke, Chapter 4, when he confronts Christ in the desert, god to god. At this point the small *s shatan* of the Old Testament becomes the capital *S* Satan, master of darkness, Lord of Hell, and in St. Matthew's anachronism, "Beelzebub the prince of the devils" (12:24). The Greco-Roman myth of Lucifer, the fallen demigod identified with the morning star, was nicely blended with this new adaptation because of a misinterpretation of Isaiah 14:12, which referred to *"Helel ben shahar,"* ("daystar, son of the dawn"). Because the daystar falls from heaven as had Lucifer, and supposedly as Satan had done, *helel* was thought to be the Greco-Roman demigod. The word *Lucifer* ("falling light" in Latin) never appears in the Hebrew Bible and is entirely a third-century A.D. accretion, derived from a classic myth.

The reinvestment of Satan (or Lucifer) fitted smoothly into pagan ideologies about demonic forces and horned deities and enabled Christianity to gain strength in Europe as well as in the Middle East. In addition, the Satan ploy fulfilled an interesting psychological need in stimulating theistic awe, for as Charles Francis Potter writes in speaking about Zoroaster, "We must admit that historically men seem to have been obliged to learn to hate the devil before they could learn to love God."[6]

Of course, countless religions existing in the first century A.D. and existing today, either have no devil of Satan's stature or regard demons as inferior to, and solely dependent on, God. Search Judaism, Islam, Buddhism, Confucianism, and even Hinduism and you'll not find a deified Satan or a Lucifer. The idea today is essentially fostered by traditional Christian theology in whatever form—whether symbolic or real—the believer chooses to believe. In the Middle Ages and early Renaissance, a very real Satan, horned, hoofed, and tailed, appeared on the scene and in the sculptured alcoves of cathedrals. The Catholics warned of him; Luther threw an inkwell at his head; Calvin skirted him at every turn; and literature abounded with his mischievous, but fascinating, personality. In most cases, Satan's presence gave meaning and merit to Christ. But, as Professor Potter again points out, there was a danger "that men may fear the devil so much that they worship him as they worship God."[7]

This they did in rituals of Satanism and witchcraft and this they do today, such as the members of La Vey's First Church of Satan headquartered in San Francisco. How ironic all this is, considering that the entity Satanists and Christians accept as a theological truth is easily traced back to the imagination of Zoroaster, blended with Greek and Roman myth and the timidities born of a shaky psychological need to explain mishap, misfortune, and death itself as something outside the pale of a merciful and saving God—and outside the pale of one's own human responsibilities. Exercising the type of casuistry such thinking inspires, Christian theologians of the Middle Ages developed the "science" of demonology in which they assigned every possible daily disorder (as they saw it) to either one demon or another. Predictably, they found the names of these demons largely in the Bible. All they had to do in this operation was to transform the ancient gods of Canaan and Philistia into monsters of depravity such as Mammon, Astarte, Beelzebub. One fifteenth-century demonologist listed 133 million such demons available to possess and destroy mankind. Each masters one or more human frailties, entering the victim through body orifices, especially during illicit sexual relations, and causing everything from vile language to putrid flatulence or amazing acrobatics. Incubi, for example, stimulate female sexual stirrings in whore and virgin alike, while succubi bring about nocturnal emissions even in the most chaste and celibate priests. (How else could you explain such things?)

## Satan Today

But that was in the Middle Ages. Do people today really believe in an anthropomorphic devil, a verifiable Satan, who rivals Christ, inspires demons, and seeks to rule the world—or in fact already rules it?

According to a poll taken in the spring of 1973, before *The Exorcist* craze, by the Center for Policy Research, 48 per cent of some 3,500 Americans questioned were certain that the devil exists. Another 20 per cent thought his existence possible. Ten years before, 37 per cent surveyed believed in a viable Satan. Clyde Z. Nunn, the director of the poll, attributed the unusual findings in 1973 to a general sense of helplessness in the world, where "things seem to be falling apart."[8]

In another poll, taken during *The Exorcist* craze (April 1974), Louis Harris found that 53 per cent of those questioned believed in the devil per se and 36 per cent in possession by the devil. Furthermore, seven million adults, said Harris, believe that someone close to them has actually been demonically possessed. Only 30 per cent of the sample polled rejected belief in a valid Satan, Lucifer, devil, demon, or whatever you want to call it.

The Evangelist Billy Graham added his voice to the majority. "I believe in the devil," he was quoted as saying, "and I believe in God, and I'm trying to get people to vote for God."[9] At the Vatican, even before *The Exorcist* was released as a film, a special declaration affirming Satan's existence was issued on the authority of Pope Paul VI. Citing biblical passages, in December 1972 the Pope stated: "We thus know that this obscure and disturbing being really exists and that he still operates with treacherous cunning; he is the occult enemy who sows errors and disgrace in human history."[10] And lest anyone assume the Pope is referring to a symbolic, allegoric conceit, he continues by personifying the fiend as a "perfidious and astute charmer, who manages to insinuate himself into us by way of the senses, of fantasy, of concupiscence, of utopian logic, of disorderly social contracts."[11] The Pope furthermore called for a reinstitution of demonology as a modern study of note.

Liberal Catholic clergy were probably caught off guard by these sacred pronouncements. The Reverend Eugene Kennedy, a psychologist at Loyola University in Chicago, was quoted in the New York *Times* as insisting that "being a Christian and a mature person means coming to terms with our own capacity for evil, not projecting it on an outside force that possesses us."[12] But his was a minority voice. In general, the Pope's declaration greatly appealed to Dualists—and exorcists—and many others who supposedly deplore the occult. Father John J. Nicola, assistant director of the National Shrine of the Immaculate Conception in Washington, D.C., and technical adviser for the exorcism scenes in *The Exorcist,* took advantage of his celebrity to assert belief in Satan, in possession, and, reiterating Baudelaire, warned that the devil's greatest weapon is the belief that he does *not* exist. Presumably, those who do not believe in him are therefore willing, or unwilling, emissaries of hell and this includes more than half the population of the world who are not fundamentalist Christians or, redundantly, Dualists.

More subtle apologists, like the Reverend Andrew M. Greeley, a Roman Catholic who is program director of the Center for the Study of American Pluralism at the National Opinion Research Center of the University of Chicago, writing in the Sunday New York *Times* of February 1973, walked an ambiguous line between the papal assertion and a form of poetic analogy. "Something," he said, is responsible for "mistakes, miscalculations . . . hurricanes, earthquakes." It is not precisely a thing called Satan, although something very much like Satan seems to be guiding it, and according to Greeley, guiding it "brilliantly."[13]

The Christian dilemma in both affirming and yet denouncing Satan is much more responsible for the current witchcraft or occultic craze than any threat of hydrogen bombs or oil embargoes. The so-called witches and Satanists I have met in the course of teaching and lecturing are largely strict observers, now lapsed, who have easily substituted Satan for Christ in adherence to an early religious indoctrination that makes it impossible for them to view the world in other than dualistic terms. Given the depth of the psychological weaknesses current today as demonstrated by the hysterical reaction to *The Exorcist,* can we afford less than a crisp, clear realization of the devil as a myth? To affirm his reality is to affirm dualism with all its hang-ups, alibis, and tendencies toward schizo-phrenic guilt. A recognition that evil is a man-made reaction, that man for all his inner torments and outer struggles, his kidnapings, hijackings, and heroin addiction would be better served by seeking to refine the difference between justice and injustice, right and wrong, seems to me to be far more useful today than all the current mythologizing in dualistic terms about good and evil.

Believing Satan responsible for hurricanes, earthquakes, sexual malaise, and every other faulty condition provides an impoverished, pessimistic view of life and stimulates irrational compulsiveness as illustrated by Captain Ahab in *Moby Dick*. At the worst it can also lead to outright murder. Samuel De Nicola in 1974 confessed to the slaying of a Long Island coed because, as he stated in court, he had "acted under orders from the devil," who was his master, who em-powered him and wished him to lead a satanic revival in the world. In his written plea, De Nicola further confessed that "what he does for Satan cannot be judged wrong, that if he murdered . . . it was to point up the frailties of a believer of Jesus Christ when met by a disciple of Satan."[14]

One of the murderers in the infamous Manson case, also known as the Sharon Tate murders, believed himself to be Satan acting out the dictum that what is evil is really good and what is good is really evil. And then there was the drowning of the baby in Manhattan (1975) by a Satan-possessed housekeeper, also acting under orders from her "god."

As stated, these are the extremes of the Dualist compulsion. The Jekyll-Hyde rationale, however, may also influence less lurid reac-tions to the general superstitious tendency now under discussion. After all, it was Dr. Jekyll himself who described a fairly common view of human dichotomy that sounds very much like Dualist reasoning: " . . . I learned to recognize the thorough and primitive duality of man," he said. "I saw that, of the two natures that con-tended in the field of my consciousness, even if I could rightly be said to be either, it was only because I was radically both."[15]

A belief that the universe is a Zoroastrian battlefield in which Satan contends with God leads to a view that the individual himself is a similar, miniature battlefield of two natures, just as Jekyll sees it. Sometimes one will have the upper hand; sometimes the other. Responsibility is beyond the subject's control. He is moral and beneficent because God wills it, or he is destructive and base because the Evil One momentarily rules. Unfortunately, as Stevenson's famous story relates, the malicious Mr. Hyde soon overtakes the worthy Dr. Jekyll, despite all his good intentions and alibis.

When the conflict born of a Dualist view is acute and enduring, a type of possession may seem to have occurred, in which an actual emissary of hell, a demon—or *the* demon—has infused the victim's body. This apprehension, glorified in *The Exorcist,* is sanctioned in modern thinking of countless biblical passages, no doubt the same ones cited by the Pope in his assertion of Satan quoted above. True, the demons who possess and cripple the bodies of New Testament characters, such as the dumb man of Matthew 9:32, have an ambiguous status in many scholarly minds. Some observers imply that they are not devils in the demonological sense, but rather closer to the concept of "unclean spirits" that the Hebrews believed caused mysterious diseases. But whatever the scholars may believe, the average Bible reader comes away from passages like Matthew 9:32 or the famous recitation about the Gadarene in Mark 5:1–9 with the belief that demon possession can and does occur as part of the God-versus-Satan battle for man's soul, that this same foreign agent can maliciously control all or part of one's personality, that it can create havoc and supernatural events, that its malice is unselective, falling on guilty and innocent alike, and that it is usually and violently unresponsive to treatment.


### *Those Possessed*


For physicians, psychiatrists, and other counselors, Satanism as a superstitious malady represents practically a dead end as far as remission is concerned. The patient beset by demonic beliefs is a schizoid locked into his dilemma by convictions, which he consciously, or unconsciously, considers fixed and righteous, willed by God or by the devil—in any event, willed by a supernatural force unyielding even to the pretensions of medicine. Has not St. Thomas Aquinas written that all mental disorder is demonic in origin, ergo curable only by prayer or exorcism?

Victims in this category of Dualist superstition—and it is a category best labeled. "Disease"—are often steeped in other irrational beliefs, such as voodoo, astrology, and so forth. They are literate in the sense of having familiarity with fantastic writings, films, and other representations of the occult, and they frequently also evince symptoms of psychosexual maladjustment and antisocial (aggressive) behavior. The favorite, often unspoken, motto of such persons is "the devil made me do it," and this covers for them a multitude of sins and personal disclaimers of responsibility for anything.

Because of the deep-seated religious beliefs that support the psychoneurosis of possession and the resulting traumas, some argue that it may be occasionally necessary to encourage an exorcism ritual on the theory that counteraction intimately related to the formation of the problem, the "possession," effectively relieves, at least initially, both the disturbance as such and, progressively, the external symptoms. I say initially because the dreaded symptoms usually return. After all, exorcism deals with demons not with disease and demons are supposed to be relentless and only temporarily offended by ritual. Since the abreaction experienced by the victim in exorcism is unrelated to the deeper causes and fallacies of his disturbance, exorcism can only function as an interim remedy, if a remedy at all. The superficial efficacy of the ritual (and I have no statistics to indicate that it is, in fact, a generally effective operation) points up the Dualist nucleus of the problem at hand, since the person possessed demonstrates by the very act of yielding up his demon, the existence of a superstitious motivation from the first. (Interestingly enough, in *The Exorcist*, the little girl who is presumably possessed and successfully exorcized is irrationally presented as being completely indifferent and ignorant where religion is concerned.) The fact is that psychologically speaking, one cannot exorcize a demon from an honest atheist because in his belief he would never be demonized to begin with. Effective, though short-term, exorcism of demon possessors can only be expected in those cases where deep-seated religious, that is Christian, views are held—and this tells us much about the situation.

A classic case of such possession (demonomania) reported by Freud in *The Interpretation of Dreams* yielded to psychotherapy and points up a variety of realistic contributory factors demonstrating that such cases are of a medical or psychiatric nature and not at all the result of some supernatural manifestation. Albert, when he was thirteen—at the onset of puberty—became subject to violent hallucinations in which the devil appeared in such vividness that the boy could actually smell the proverbial pitch and brimstone of hell and feel the fire singeing his skin. The hallucination occurred in tandem with masturbatory experiments and were so intensely fearful that Albert avoided undressing "because the fire attacked him only when he was undressed." The analyst on the case drew the following profile of the unfortunate boy:

1) He was physically weak, suffering from cerebral anemia possibly attributed to heredity and a syphilitic condition in his father.

2) The anemia produced an alteration of character, which triggered, via brain chemistry, demonic hallucinations and dreams.

3) The choice of the demonic trauma resulted from the influences of childhood religious education vis-à-vis the evils of masturbation and the horrors of hell.

In short, physical predisposition (cerebral anemia), plus the stress of puberty (masturbation guilt), caused the negative reaction in the form of a mental disease.


## Universal Exorcism


Given the widespread dissemination of superstitious ideas about possession these days, Christian upbringing or belief may not be necessary for the adverse Dualist reaction. A half-page ad in New York's *Village Voice* in the spring of 1974 was a dubious lesson-at-a-glance about the subject, warning that "possession of the mind and body by evil spirits can happen to anyone, anywhere, any time. It is a universal state, common to all religions and beliefs, to all places and periods of history . . ."[16]

The point of the ad was to hustle talismans and an LP record of the Roman Catholic exorcism ritual. The alleged universality of the possession phenomenon was further plugged by an offering of "sacred spells, objects and rituals feared by the Devil in Jewish, as well as Catholic and Indian rituals . . ."[17]

Jewish beliefs in possession, which are extrabiblical, do not concern demons, since Judaism eschews a Satan figure, but rather involve spirits of the undead, *dybbuks*, who, in legend, seek to enter the body of a loved one or kin. A Yiddish play, *The Dybbuk*, written in the 1900s, represents almost the total extent of knowledge on this peripheral myth. Nevertheless, modern-day Jews who want to be hip can talk themselves into dybbuk-possession as easily as Christians may open themselves to demonic blandishments. The bugaboos are indeed universal, as proved in the case of a Jewish boy named Jake, age fourteen, who was apparently cognizant enough of Dualist superstition to be afflicted by what he called a "stuttering devil," that is, a devil that caused him to stutter. As reported by Dr. Herbert A. Aikins, Jake would often be visited in his dreams or in his thoughts by a certain "greenish-black" creature with horns and the wings of a bat, something like the fiend that confronted Martin Luther. This past association demonstrated Jake's wide reading in religious fields. He knew from such investigations that being Jewish he could not protect himself from Satan by making the sign of the cross. So like Luther, Jake tried to throw an inkwell at his supposed enemy.

Under psychoanalysis, the stutterer began to associate the demon with a mad dog who had chased him when he was five years old, an incident that brought on the first bout of stuttering. Jake believed the ghost of this dog, who was killed in front of his eyes, was tangibly haunting him in the devilish form. After extensive recall, the patient finally made a breakthrough when he grew to realize that his fear of the dog, disguised as a devil, was the root of his stuttering symptoms. Dr. Aikins described his treatment, which eventually cured the boy, as a "breaking up" of the emotional habit or reaction symptomized by stuttering. By drawing Jake back to the source of the habit (the mad dog), he was "encouraging him to stop and examine each spooky object [of the habit] until nameless fear gives way to confident knowledge . . . This is breaking up the habit from within."[18]

The religious ritual of exorcism and other similar panderings to demonic ideas only reinforce the spookiness of each object, do nothing to break them up from within, and therefore are likely to guarantee relapse and repetition of the traumas involved.

The Dualist trend, as noted, is not limited to the United States. A Toronto newspaper early in 1975 reported the "growing popularity" of exorcism across Canada, adding "what was considered an uncommon practice has now almost become common, and this is even more true in the United States and Britain where . . . the press pays no attention to it anymore."[19] The Canadian trend is a distinctly Protestant undertaking, according to this report.

In England, a certain Anglican minister has been exorcizing the demon-ridden of his parish since 1949, and according to the *Wall Street Journal*, "following the appearance of the Blatty book and movie, [the exorcisms] have escalated up to 10 a week . . ."

Throughout Great Britain, the *Journal* goes on, there is a surge of "requests to drive away demons, ghosts and poltergeists not only from traditionally haunted castles, but also from crowded pubs and brand-new apartments."[20]

Commenting on the craze, the conservative British paper the *Sunday Telegraph*, plunging through the Dualist trap, acknowledged that dwelling on evil spirits "could degenerate into a grisly superstition," but quickly added, "we should be rash to go to the other extreme and assume that there are no devils in London."[21]

Considering that England is rife with self-proclaimed witches, mediums, and occultniks of all varieties, numbering, according to one estimate, some three million individuals, and given the ostensible sanction of the Anglican church regarding devils and ghosts, is it any wonder that along with its general political decline, Great Britain may now be the foremost battlefield of Dualist superstition outside of Los Angeles? The Anglican exorcizer referred to above is well aware of this but views the English situation in clear-cut Dualist terms as a battle between the witches and the church. "Large numbers of people have been bewitched," he claims, and cannot resume normal activities until exorcized. But Richard Janssen, who wrote the *Wall Street Journal* article, quite astutely sees something else slinking within the British psyche, which he calls "a longing for a spark of mystery in a Christianity that has been largely drained of angels and hellfire."[22] In a phrase, it is the Dualist superstition of angels and hellfire, Satan versus God, that is pervasively making itself felt like the London fog.

## Myth and Misrepresentation

The development of myths is a study in itself and an exhausting one. For our purposes, it should be noted that myths often arise from specific cultures in order to fulfill specific explanatory needs. When myths are believed in religious or quasi-religious terms, we are then faced with a form of superstition, such as outlined in the case of demon possession.

Granted, there is a place for myth in life. Its function in aid of fantasy and as escapist fare is well regarded by psychologists, and the mythical basis of much art and drama is often stimulating. In these positive cases, myth is understood to be myth, not divine utterance, not unalterable truth, or, worse yet, proof.

The negative function of myth derives from an ironic situation. Because they are born of particular cultures and specific, often forgotten, needs, myths can become distorted in readaptation. Relying on them in such cases is like swallowing other people's medicines, prescribed for their maladies and their needs but possibly dangerous for ours. Satan is a myth of this negative sort simply because he falls into certain myth-structure definitions and specific cultural origins.

The myth of Satan does not militate against the reality of evil men and wicked deeds or certain actual occurrences that people reckon as satanic in nature. In such cases, a small *s* satanic is a useful unanthropormorphic synonym for the annoyingly inexplicable. Nor are we rushing in with a sledgehammer to beat off the fleas by asserting that Satan, capital S, is totally functionless in allegoric terms. As a figure in art, particularly in Milton's *Paradise Lost*, he is a grand and welcome creation, and how better to describe Hitler than in capital S Satanist vocabulary? But as the other side of the cosmic coin, as rival to an elevated view of God, a viable Satan has the negative function of transforming that God into a comparable myth and popular religion into a horror show.

Some might say the opposite—that debunking Satan, depropagandizing his reality, does precisely the same for God. You can't have one without the other, and conversely, if Satan is a myth, why not Yaweh (or Jehovah) or Christ? Here is where some eggshell walking takes place, and yet, the challenge is welcomed, even though it be briefly met. By tracing the origin, development, and current status of the biblical figure Jehovah, we may very well come to agree that it is a myth, formed by men and traceable in Semitic ideology, and that Jesus Christ of Nazareth is an euhemeristic idea, at best, meaning that he may have been a real man transformed into a god, or, as Albert Schweitzer believed, "the Jesus of Nazareth who came forth publicly as the Messiah . . . never had any existence . . ."[23] The spiritual Jesus, the God before human manufacturing, however, is a very real entity in Schweitzer's view. The same may be said of God per se, God the transcendent deity, whose origins are everywhere and nowhere, whose development is not a progressive line, but rather a circle and one "without circumference," to quote St. Bonaventura. As regards tangents and ornaments, God is continually being adorned *and* divested of them, now as in the past. His current status is therefore beside the point and, in so being, he achieves a position unlike any other myth or reality. In short, by the cherished tenets of ontological proof, God seems outside any one man's brain, unrelated to a specific culture, undeveloped from any singular drawing board, as much a mystery in current status as in ages past—and mystery is not synonymous with myth—and probably a noumenon more than a phenomenon, and a noumenon that is obviously impenetrable by man.

So much for circular proofs (if they *are* proofs); the point here is to place Satan in perspective and vitiate the dualism that weighs so greatly in modern superstitious thought. Unfortunately, with the Bible functioning in part, to many, as a sort of occultic Baedeker, a popular rational as opposed to Dualist view in religious terms seems increasingly remote, and so it shall remain until the Bible reader remembers the more philosophical, the more humane, the more insightful passages of that amazing document. Remembers the warning in Jeremiah concerning the general problem of mythic and occultic deceits: "The prophets prophesy lies in my name; I sent them not . . . they prophesy unto you a false vision and divination, and a thing of nought, and the deceit of their heart" (14:14).

At this point, I imagine some may say, smirking with Shakespeare, that "the devil can cite Scripture for his purpose," which may be true if the devil were real. Ah, but then, recalling Baudelaire and C. S. Lewis, to boot, the same smirker may retort that it is the devil's delight to be disproven and that they who do so work on his behalf since he likes us to be unguarded in thinking he is merely a fairy tale.

Believing Mickey Mouse to be a myth, I hope it will not also be said of me, in this vein, that I am in the service of Walt Disney—or Donald Duck. Actually, I view myself closer to the famous words of St. John: "Ye shall know the truth, and the truth shall make you free."

That too is from the Bible.

CHAPTER 3

# Wolf's Tooth, Cross, and Peperone

In the thirteenth-century conjurer's book known as the *Clavicule de Salomon*, one may read of a talisman for resisting the attacks of evildoers, which, according to one source, enables you when armed with it to "venture during the most advanced hours of the night into the most cut-throat and ill-famed quarters of the capitals of the five divisions of the globe." This talisman is so powerful, the description continues, that the possessor if "attacked by any man shall not be hurt by him or wounded when [he] fights with him . . ."[1]

In the 1970s, an advertisement appeared in the Sunday New York *Times* for a talisman of love, similarly, and allegedly, derived from the magic lore of Solomon, which when worn as a pendant may "invoke response in love, personal favor and passion . . . a symbol of deep affection and a promise of true love."

One should note the more ambiguous promises of the twentieth-century offering as compared to the thirteenth-century charm, although recent claims for copper armbands and elephant-hair bracelets are, in fact, more egregious in stipulating revitalized health, youthful sex, and general good fortune. But no matter which century offers the most, clearly there is still today—as there has always been—an abiding fascination and belief in the ancient superstition of sympathetic magic, that is, the notion that wearing or possessing certain items and objects somehow provides the owner with specific doses of luck and success (or his enemy with the opposite). Because King Solomon, whom occultists regard as a wondrous seer, allegedly devised or wore such talismans himself, and because these talismans were engraved with ancient mantic symbols and signs, we may expect a sort of unmeasurable radiation to emanate from any reproductions of the original and thereby re-establish the original protective impulse. The two separate triangles of the six-pointed star (Shield of David or Seal of Solomon), the talismans mentioned above, reportedly symbolize fire and water, God and man, male and female, and several other opposite attractions. Combined, they must logically represent a sort of locked-in power or force drawing from each extreme; protective against maliciousness in one case (the alliance of God and man—an unbeatable combo) and in the other, stimulating love as a result of the overlapping of the male and female (which, we presume, is the aim of the love talisman in the first place).

In most cases where charms, amulets, talismans, lucky colors, clothing, perfumes, and so forth are worn (or possessed) in superstitious terms, the wearer is seeking some form of easily won success or protection and may therefore be motivated by any number of superstitious ideologies: appeasement, expiation, dualism, and so forth. Because he interprets these ideas in a tangible way, a psychological implication may be drawn about specific physical insecurities. The wearers of lucky colors, for instance, may believe themselves homely or bodily unattractive; talismans, especially in the form of pendants, may indicate a socio-sexual hang-up; possession of charmed items, fetishes, or amulets, may unconsciously symbolize inhibitions regarding person-to-person contact, the holder of the charm preferring to caress its allegedly magical surface rather than the body of another human being. Fascination or obsession with tangible aspects of superstition usually originates in the realms of physical consideration, bodily protection, or expression. In some cases, however, the superstition is one step removed as the individual transfers the particular talisman or amulet from his own body to that of his surroundings (house, car, bedstead). Taken as a whole, these objects and items may be called trinkets—tangible aspects of superstition—and the type of people who rely on them, in whatever degree, referred to as Trinketeers.


## A Catalogue of Trinkets


Superstitious affection for objects, a belief in their magical powers, is possibly as old as man's ability to grasp a stick, a stone, or some fragment of an animal bone. Studies of chimpanzees today indicate their instincts for holding objects and waving them at enemies, just as early man may have shaken a branch at a thundering sky in the hopes of altering its effect. The magic wand, or stick, is therefore one of the earliest occultic objects we find in primitive use. Its visual relation to the phallus (also believed then, as now, to possess magical powers) doubles its power as a superstitious archetype. In this vein, the iron wand or spear of Mars is considered an object of fertility and is visualized in astronomy by the symbol,

$$\mathlarge{\male}$$

which is also the sign of the male.

From Neanderthal graves we note that teeth and bone fragments may have been believed to have magical powers, since both were ceremoniously buried with the dead, possibly as propitiatory small change for a life beyond. Such items were technically amulets, or natural trinkets in their natural forms. Far more popular is the category of trinkets known as talismans, a word originating in the Greek *telesma,* meaning something of a sacred and also manufactured origin, a consecrated device which may be worn, nailed to a wall, or hung around a cradle. In most cases, talismans are constructed for protective purposes, like the one from the *Clavicule de Salomon.* They often have ceremonial or attractive functions as well in the sense of attracting beneficent forces, specifically sexual love.

The makers of talismans, occultists by definition, believed effective devices of this sort must be fashioned under proper magical conditions, during astrologically sanctioned periods, and wrought of materials which have supposedly magical properties in and of themselves (like parchment, precious gems, or bone). Talismans differ from amulets by virtue of their ceremonial manufacture. The cross carved out of bone is talismanic, while the bone worn as is may be defined as an amulet—a charm devised from a natural object, which retains its natural condition with only the slightest alteration, if any.

By and large, religious adornments and jewelry are talismanic in origin. The most popular of these are the crucifix; the cross; the Jewish star; the ankh; the Hebrew chai; the tiki; and specific saint medallions, usually worn by Catholics. All may be classified, if superstitiously worn, as trinkets. Each deserves a bit of separate investigation considering their popularity in modern times.


### The Cross and Crucifix


Centuries before the Christian Era, the cross was a common device and symbol indicative of the four geographic poles or of an outstretched man. Seen as an X, it also symbolized the axis of the universe and slightly crooked, with right-angle hooks on each leg, it appears as the swastika, a Hindu solar sign in use long before its adaption and debasement by the Nazi party.

Carl Gustav Jung regards the world-wide appearance of the cross in any form, even as an architectural ground plan, as an expression of "the deepest insights of consciousness and the loftiest intuitions of the spirit, thus amalgamating the uniqueness of present-day consciousness and the age-old past of humanity."[2] Jung further relates this symbol to fire since two sticks rubbed together, crosswise, were used by primitive man to produce a flame and with it "magic." Less romantic views of the cross include its function, even today, as the signature of an illiterate, who usually makes his "mark" with an X or a cross because such marks are among the simplest to draw and are therefore often found in basic pottery designs as well as doodling. Of course, there are many reinterpretations even of the simple cross; among them the elaborate Christian crucifix, the truncated tau or T cross, the ansate cross (or ankh), the papal cross with its three vertical bars, or the modern peace cross, which looks like an inverted Y in a circle. Of them all, only the Christian forms seem inclined in magical paths, that is, in purely protective, scare-away-devils functions, and the idea behind this no doubt developed from specific pagan usage of the symbol. We know the Druids of Celtic Europe employed a cross as a symbol for consecrational rites related to the moon and the four poles. Druid-Christian intercourse was sufficiently common by the third or fourth centuries A.D. for various aspects of the pagan cult to drift unnoticed into Christian art and ritual. The druidic Queen of Heaven, for example, became the prototype of Regina Coeli (Mary, Queen of Heaven); Druid mistletoe evolved as a Christmas symbol; the celebration of All Saints' Day (November 1) seems to have been inspired by the Celtic Allhallows' Eve (October 31)—and so forth. In any event, the magical, talismanic powers of the cross or crucifix in Christianity, as we know it, did *not* originate with the early followers of Christ in the Middle East. They at first employed the Greek letter chi (X) as a secret sign of their cult. To them it signified the first letter of the word Christ and was in no way mantic. Adding the R, or rho, gave these early worshipers the symbol,

$$\text{☧}$$

chi-rho. This was a call-letter sign, not a talisman, nor did it symbolize the crucifixion. Besides, the early Christians were all faithful Jews, who were prohibited by commandment from adorning themselves in any device or geometric symbol that could be taken for representations of either gods or men.

Centuries later, when the Church Fathers of Europe wished to win pagan souls to Christ, they encouraged converts, especially of the Celtic regions, to regard the cross as a symbol of Christ in tandem with their own druidic device. Before long, the pagan practice of wearing talismans (i.e., the cross around the neck) became a Christian tradition. Elaborations of the cross then followed, continually falling back on mantic and idolatrous concepts of talismans. This is particularly evident when the body of Christ was superimposed on the cross, hence the crucifix, making it a later-day development of fertility poles used in Rome to glorify Attis, the chief Asiatic resurrection god. At the vernal equinox, well into Christian times, an effigy of Attis in an ithyphallic condition was displayed nailed or tied to a portable tree trunk—the modern derivative of which has come to be the Maypole. In some cases, according to Frazer, the tree itself was transformed into a "corpse," by being swathed in bloodstained woolen bands.[3] A young pagan god on a tree, or cross, turned into a corpse and employed for fertility or magical rites is the actual origin of the Christian crucifix and has nothing to do with the biblical Christ, per se.

In the seventh century A.D. at Trullo, the Church finally officialized the crucifix, therefore the cross, making it a holy emblem and thus, by extrapolation, a talismanic device. Trinketeers today regard it primarily in this fashion and many believe that it can ward off demons, vampires, satanic influences, and all the miseries they portend. This is especially true if the cross is "flashed" or held up ritualistically, as the celebrant does at the Mass. The offending forces will then fall back before the symbol of the crucified Jesus, whether it is an actual jewel-encrusted cross on a pole, a small crucifix on a necklace, or the cruciform hilt of a sword. Lacking these, the protective sign may be created by superimposing the index fingers of each hand one over the other. A simpler and more common form of this improvised propitiation—and one that has come to represent "good luck" and the anticipation of good fortune—is the act of twisting the index finger and the middle finger of the right hand one over the other in remembrance of the Crucifixion.

Oddly enough, in recent times, the pagan origins of the cross have become more apparent as Christian Trinketeers feel it necessary to bolster "crucial" powers with other talismans in close proximity. A fabricated piece of coral or gold in the shape of the horn or pepper is commonly seen dangling alongside the crucifix these days, blending two ancient superstitions in a revealing way.

## The Star or Shield of David

As just noted, religious Jews do not approve of any articles that can be taken as deferences to idolatry. Consequently, Orthodox people today will not wear any jewelry or insignia that may be regarded as talismanic. Even so, the trinketeering instinct is as strong among modern Jews as it is among any other group and as a result, a plethora of trinkets may be found around Jewish necks, including the Star of David, the mezuzah, the letter chai, the horns, Zodiac signs, St. Christopher medals, and the like.

The Star of David, or hexagram, was specifically talismanic even before its adoption into Jewish lore, which seems to have been fairly late in the post-Christian Era. No mention of the *Magen David* (Shield or Star of David) can be found in the Old Testament or in rabbinic literature, and it is believed to have first been associated with Jews in second-century B.C. Greece, where the letter delta

$$(\triangle)$$

stood for David; two deltas superimposed were an abbreviation of the ancient King's full name.

As elemental symbols, the two triangles from which the star is made, one on its apex, the other on its base, represent fire and water and were used as such in medieval alchemy. Gnostics and magicians of this period, especially those who dabbled in kabala, regarded the fusing of the two signs as an act of magic and created from it the "Seal of Solomon," identical in design to the Star of David but unrelated in Judaic tradition. It was this seal which they used as a protective symbol when conjuring demons, and it became the essential design in elaborate talismans, such as the one referred to at the opening of this chapter.

Combining opposites as the star seems to do (fire-water, man-God, male-female, et cetera) supposedly empowers any talisman with unearthly effects. But this does not automatically make the Star of David a historical talisman. In fact, among Jews it is primarily a patriotic insignia and as such was adopted by the First

Zionist Congress in 1897 as the emblem of the Jewish state, where today it appears on flags and stamps. (The official seal of the State of Israel, by the way, is a seven-branched candelabrum or Menorah.)

The Seal of Solomon is quite a different story. It is, despite its biblical name, a *non*-Jewish symbol as described above. Modern Jews who wear the hexagram, therefore, have to face the following dilemma: if they wear it as a talisman, then it is not Judaic (rather it is pagan and medieval, possibly even Christian, in the sense of Gnostic). If worn as a badge of Judaism, it is in no way religious or magical, but rather historical. The only specific Judaic talisman, sanctioned by rabbis and mentioned indirectly in the Bible, is the mezuzah, or doorpost talisman, which contains a piece of scroll with excerpts from Deuteronomy, Chapters 6–11 handwritten on it. Though frequently worn around the neck on a chain, the mezuzah is not intended to be a bodily charm and therefore will be discussed later under household talismans.

## *Life Signs*

Two symbols or alphabetic representations of the word "life" are now commonly worn on chains apparently for talismanic purposes, though one may suspect that they are really more the invention of Trinketeers than the result of either Jungian or cultural reality. In addition, it seems as though one, the ankh, led to the other, the chai.

The ankh

☥

is sometimes called the ansate cross and was thought to be a Greek derivative in which a tau or T cross, representing "life," was surmounted with a circle, representing "eternity." The implication was "the life to come" or eternal life. The figure, however, was actually adopted by the Greeks from Pharaonic Egypt, where it was, in hieroglyphs, the sound *ankh* and, coincidentally, the ancient word for "life." Symbolized, the ankh appears in many Egyptian bas-reliefs as an object carried by the gods, particularly Isis, who, as the guardian of medicine, invests it with the meaning of health. The eternal-life connotation as well as principles of male-female, above-below, and man-god are also believed imparted by this word-sign.

As an actual talisman, one intended to produce a magical effect, the ankh, as I have mentioned, is more the product of the Trinketeer than it is of ancient sorcery. Psychologically, it may function as a symbol that nicely breaks with tradition (i.e., the Christian cross) and goes back to the so-called "source" (ancient Egypt) for the ultimate magical impact.

In Hebrew, the word for "life" is *chai* (we are all familiar with the Jewish toast *L'chayim*, "to our lives.") Spelled out in Hebrew letters,

חי

the word has become a sort of Judaized ankh and is worn on chains, rings, and imprinted as a talismanic, or at least propitiatory, design. Again, there is nothing in Judaism to support usage of the chai for any "supernatural" purposes. It is purely a gimmick and has no history as a talisman, even in kabala.


### Tikis, Jujus, and Fish


The tendency among Trinketeers to research ancient and culturally foreign objects for veneration has been touched on in relation to the ankh. Popular in this category as well, are exotic talismans such as the tikis from Polynesia, of which Kon-Tiki is perhaps the most famous. The Hei-Tiki is actually the one considered magical by the Maori of New Zealand. Like all tikis, it is a phallic representation of man, in this case the world's first man, who was fashioned in this shape by the gods themselves. Hei-Tiki is intended to be worn around the neck as a stimulus to fertility.

The fish is another popular piece of exotica worn on chains and usually made of several parts so that it undulates like a fish or like the phallus, which it probably represented in pagan minds. As a symbol of Christ, the fish derives from ICHTHUS, the Greek word for fish, which when taken as an acrostic means, "Jesus Christ, Son of God, Saviour of Men." Because of this association, the fish is also popular, especially among fishing peoples, as a talisman related to the crucifix.

From Polynesia come various tikis or talismans, many of which are spurious, adapted from the originals to appeal to ethnic rather than mantic needs. Included with these are the jujus or African tribal talismans in the forms of snakes, hands, tikilike figures, and other natural objects. Often these are carved in ebony.

## Gems and Beads

The talismanic reputation of certain gems opens up a treasure chest of superstitious inclinations, one, happily, replete with lovely objects which regale the eye despite any magical needs or expectations. A language of jewels has arisen since kabalistic times which implies that one may wear a certain gem to achieve a certain protective end. Thus, pearls, because of their moonlike look, are recommended as talismanic adornments for women during menstrual (or moon) cycles; jade was thought protective against kidney disorders, possibly because it resembles kidney stones; and one report tells of a star sapphire being hawked in Thailand as the ultimate protection against "the end of the world."

Beads, being surrogates of jewels, are more accessible for magical purposes and in recent years the wearing of talismanic—as opposed to purely decorative—beads, has taken hold among the young, male and female alike. Most major religions utilize some form of rosary or string of beads as a mnemonic for prayer. Marco Polo tells of those he saw in Malabar. In fact, the English word for bead derives from *Gebet* in German (to pray) and *bede* (prayer) in Anglo-Saxon. The crudest form of the rosary, or praying beads, was a knotted string. Sikhs refer to God as "the string, the knots, the chief bead . . ." Such things developed into elegantly carved rosewood (hence rosary) beads in the Middle Ages and to necklaces of similar design in recent times. One might say that the superstitious aspect of such beads derives from early European misconceptions. Seeing Muslims and Orientals fondling beads in prayer caused observers to assume that an act of pagan (ergo effective) magic was taking place; the beads thereby adopted talismanic attributes.

## Necklaces Ad Infinitum

Wearing coins on necklace chains goes back to classic times when Roman emperors were considered sacred. Possessing their images emblazoned on coins afforded protection and demonstrated true respect since the individual preferred to venerate his emperor rather than spend his coin. Religious medals or medallions derive from this same superstitious belief. Most worn by Catholics today are coinlike in shape and design and made of metals such as silver or bronze, which, according to believers, in themselves have protective powers. Silver, like the moon, has healing potentials and frightens demons (remember the silver bullet employed to destroy werewolves). The faces or figures of saints as well as of Christ and the Virgin are represented on these talismans; St. Christopher, who has been dropped from the ranks of bona-fide Christian saints, is the most popular of these because he reportedly protects travelers, including those who drive in automobiles.

Perhaps second only to the wearing of crosses as emblems or talismans is the wearing of Zodiac signs, wrought in gold or plastic, modernized or in traditional dimensions. Whichever he chooses, the wearer implies a superstitious belief in the powers of the stars (see Chapter 6) and more so in the particular beneficent vibrations of his own special birthday period. All twelve signs are considered charged with an energy of sorts, but they are effective only if properly applied. The figures of the Zodiac are, of course, ancient gods or godly creatures like the Ram of the Golden Fleece, or Venus and Cupid transformed into the Pisces. They subsequently relate to Roman mystery religions and to their Mesopotamian forebears. Few who wear the Goat of Capricorn today realize that it is a symbol of Pan, and the panic cults—but as is true of most talismans and amulets—in fact most objects sought by the Trinketeer—the real or original meaning has been lost and only the habit is observed.

For those who wish to be fully protected in their talismanic confusion, a jeweler in California recently advertised the *dernier cri* of quasi-religious, quasi-magical adornments. It is a pendant, on a chain, about one inch in size, which combines all the major emblems dear to the hearts of Trinketeers: the ankh, which is also the cross, whose vertical bar forms part of the Star of David and supports, as well, on one arm a Muslim calligraph of Allah and, on the other, the yin and yang of oriental philosophy. Dangling below these latter symbols is an object not too easily discerned, composed of a crescent and something that looks like a turtle. Possibly it is one of those mystical composites, so loved by Jung, in which one sees whatever he wants to see: diabolic, angelic, or none of these.

### Household Luck

In referring earlier to the mezuzah, it was noted that some talismans may be affixed to one's surroundings for "luck" (i.e., protection, health, sexual success, or money). This is true of amulets as well, those *natural* objects believed to possess intrinsic powers. Among these we may list the common cluster of garlic cloves and various flowers and plants in wreaths or bouquets. Before considering the origins and meanings of these, however, we should examine the mezuzah again and with it the general and ancient concern with doorways and barriers.

To the average person, a door knocker is merely a utilitarian object, hopefully imposed with some artistic design. But, in fact, the angel's head or lion's head or certain abstract forms that we often see on doors these days are descendants of gargoyle-like artifacts intended to perform a sort of sympathetic magic in reverse. The idea is essential to any discussion of protective trinkets and superstitious psychology. Our forebears, it seems, believed that evil forces were repelled either by godly influence or by the minions of hell themselves. The theory developed that Satan feared, and still fears above all else, his own image or color (red); hence, the tying of a red ribbon to a baby's crib or the wearing of a red pepper or coral stick resembling the devil's horns or tail and thus empowered to frighten him away.

Doorways, gates, arches, windows, any orifice of a home or sacred precinct—any body orifice as well—were deemed fair game for the entrance of demons who function best when enclosed under a roof. Elaborate carvings on oriental portals are no more decorative than the gargoyles on Notre Dame de Paris, and though few of us grow geraniums in window boxes for protective purposes, our superstitious ancestors did precisely this and more: the hot red color of geraniums is admirable as a defensive row at any window, especially the kitchen, which was a favorite haunt of hellish beasts who instinctively sought out the warming fires of the hearth or stove.

Garlic is an admirable trinket for barriers given its pungent scent and horn-shaped cloves. Clusters of this common plant can still be seen nailed to doorjambs and bouqueted in kitchens. Extremist Trinketeers also adorn themselves in cloves (necklace fashion) as protection against vampires, who are particularly revulsed by the odor and shape.

The most common trinketlike device favored in America for doorway purposes is the horseshoe, which has many symbolic qualities that give comfort to superstitious fears; its hornlike shape (when properly nailed curve side downward), its metallic nature—the demon fears iron (Mars)—and the general association with the friendly horse, which misanthropic witches eschew in favor of brooms. Then there is the tale of St. Dunstan, the blacksmith, who found himself faced one day by a customer bundled in a cloak, who required reshoeing not for his horse but for himself. The smithy recognized Satan at once, remembering that the fiend, because of his cloven hoofs, often required shoeing like any dray horse. Heroic to the last, Dunstan nailed Satan to the wall and kept poking him with his red-hot tongs (fearful diabolic things even to Satan) until the demon promised never to enter any home protected by an inverted horseshoe, such as the one he so sorely craved.

This brings us back to the mezuzah, which for all its biblical sanctity is nevertheless a doorway talisman. Usually, mezuzahs are made of hollow metal tubes (metal is always protective) in which is inserted a roll of parchment properly inscribed with the Sh'ma, the central monotheistic avowal of Judaism, the words of which God commanded shall be written "upon the posts of thy house and on thy gates" (Deut. 6:9). This same Sh'ma is often regarded as a mantic invocation by magically-oriented Jews (Kabalists, for example), and because of it, the mezuzah is invested with superstitious significance. Of course, the item must be "kosher," that is pure and authentic and properly handwritten by a devout scribe on parchment without corrections or erasures. Printed scrolls inserted in the tubes are considered worthless, especially by the Lubavitcher sect of Brooklyn, New York which has recently undertaken a street campaign, with leaflets, to warn fellow Jews of impure mezuzahs being unscrupulously sold (and in the large part, those commonly sold in stores for doorways or wearing purposes are indeed "impure," i.e., unprotective).

A version of the mezuzah is the tefillin, or phylacteries, another ancient talisman also derived from Deuteronomy, where it says of the Sh'ma "and thou shalt bind [it] for a sign upon thine hand and [it] shall be as frontlets between thine eyes"; hence the small boxes, in which the same kosher scrolls are encased, held to the forehead and left upper arm (the heart line) by leather thongs during the morning prayers of pious Jews.

## Horn, Tail, and Hoof

The foregoing—the horseshoe, mezuzah, door knocker, gateway carving, and also the hex signs painted on Pennsylvania barns—must be considered talismanic since they are manufactured and not in their strictly natural form (although the horseshoe is "natural" when worn by the horse). Garlic, however, and geraniums and a host of other natural entities serve as amulets on the basis of ancient animistic ideas which invested a sort of spirit or soul (Jung would say "anima") in the most ordinary, lifeless object. For this reason, even a stone may be protective, especially a gem, like a ruby, which seems to have locked a bit of eternal fire in its depths. Being red, it is also a fearful thing for demons. This is true of the hot red pepper, the pimento, or peperone (the final "e" is usually dropped in speech), favored by Sicilian and other Italian Trinketeers as an amulet worn on the person or nailed to the house. Oddly enough, in modern times, this quintessential device has undergone a glamorous transformation that renders it almost totally useless for protective purposes. By definition, a true peperon' amulet should be a natural, dried, red vegetable, or at least a piece of red coral cut like a wiggle or pepper (horn and tail). Coral, after all, is believed to be a natural protective substance in itself. But red plastic peppers, and worse yet, gold (not even red) variations are without a shred of true trinketeering power. True, the gold variety does have the value of being metal (and a precious metal at that), but it would hardly fool any fiend unless worn in tandem with the cross, which these days it often is. (Paganism will out.)

Horn-shaped coral (the *cornuto*), often resembling an inverted Y, must also be bona fide and not plastic, so that the resemblance to the devil's horns or hoofs, coupled with the age-old veneration for coral (a Venus symbol), is rendered to the fullest effect.

## Mandrake and Other Charms

Another natural item, which, because of its shape and putative properties, has amulet value, is the mandrake root or mandragora, a much-favored item in biblical times and also in the Middle Ages. The root of a good specimen of this herb (*Mandragora officinarum*) may resemble a human figure (there are in magic terminology both male and female varieties) and thus implies certain divine considerations. When properly prepared, the herb has residual narcotic effects and, in large doses, may be poisonous. Aphrodisiac side effects have been noted as well and it is said, among believers in such things, that a test of love is to wear the obnoxious stem around one's neck; it will repel all persons save the heart's desire. In seeking mandrake, one must take very special care since it invariably brings death to those who carelessly uproot it (or so we are told). In order to prevent this fate, the seeker is advised to lasso the leafy overgrowth with a cord and then tie the free end of the cord around the neck of a dog. Tempting the animal with food, will cause him, not you, to uproot the plant and promptly fall dead as a result. (Reportedly, the shriek emitted by the mandrake as it is unearthed causes death to the unearther.)

Clearly, form and effect have played their parts in making substances like pepper, coral, mandrake, and even human bones magical in amulet terms. There are other such items, however, that appeal for less obvious reasons, among them the rabbit's foot (which one must consider an amulet owing to its natural form), the four-leafed clover, human hair, teeth, and representations of the hand. The latter, though reproduced, should be regarded as "natural" since we do not want to encourage amputation of real hands even for the high and mighty purposes of trinketeering.

The rabbit's foot, or paw, is thought effective as a fertility and luck symbol. Rabbits are synonymous with fertility and as a result of their rapid breeding are often slaughtered as pests, thus providing plenty of paws. Certain ancient totem ideas may be vested in this and all other animal amulets (monkey's paws, tiger's claws, et cetera). Primitive man believed, with a sort of pre-Darwinian insight, that he had ascended from lowly animals, the rabbit and mouse among them. Animal veneration was in part the result of this conceit, and totem poles, especially as carved by American Indians, duly represent the upward climb from simple beast, at the bottom, to full-formed man. Rather than carry around a whole totem pole, or the dried-up rabbit as such, men decided on the paw as a useful pendant and commonly wear or carry one even to this day.

Hands or paws are, after all, rather magical in themselves, considering their powers and impetus to human development. Without our functioning hands, many anthropologists believe we would still be prosimians crouching dumbly in trees. The Hand of God, the Hand of Fate, various finger positions (or mudras), may be considered amulets when worn as charms or pendants, even if reproduced in metal or some other substance. The actual hand, alive and well in its proper place, serves admirably as a protective device (and I don't refer here to its pugilistic potentials). By forming certain modern mudras, the Trinketeer can effect desired results with a veritable flick of the wrist. We have already mentioned crossing the fingers as a hasty, last-ditch crucifix sign; in addition, one may "flash" the horns to scare devils, by extending the little finger and index finger while lowering the other two fingers and thumb. This "flash" must be done with the palm forward, toward the antagonist. The palm facing the flasher causes the mudra to imply cuckoldry—and worse. Inserting the thumb between the clenched index finger and its neighbor, signals "a fig on you" (or worse) and is useful for scaring fiends, who hate the fecundity seedy figs connote. Then there is the phallic thrust: middle finger erect, all others folded, clearly offensive to life-hating fiends.

The hair of the head is no less magical than the hand and available as an amulet per se, especially a curl or braid embedded in a locket or brooch. The origins of this practice go back to the veneration of the head discussed in Chapter 1. As an outgrowth of that sacred dome, hair seemed impregnated with the bearer's soul. For this reason it can be wickedly used by voodoo practitioners who append it to their fearsome pin-stuck dolls. But ladies of the chivalric age were romantic, not wicked, and when they snipped a curl for a knight, they did so as an act of fealty; the soul was literally surrendered in a lock of hair and according to Alexander Pope, in his *Rape of the Lock*, "mighty contests rise from [such] trivial things." Many peoples keep such relics of deceased loved ones, or pets, in the belief that something of the person remains in the tresses. Such in fact is the premise of all religious relics, which are often viewed as talismanic, or more accurately, amuletic wonderments.

Teeth, human and animal, have a weighty folklore surrounding them, since they appear to be uncanny organs, unlike any other in the body. Consider: which other part of us is absent at birth but then "grows" in and once having grown, falls out only to be replaced? Teeth are often regarded as omens and certain aborigines, it is said, will kill a child whose uppers erupt before his lowers, for fear that the child will get the "upper" hand—or more precisely the "upper bite"—on things. Canine teeth in some places are feared, which is natural considering their ferocious appearance in the mouth of a wolf or tiger (or vampire). When the animal is subdued, the canine is often extracted for amulet purposes; it will impart courage and strength, give the bearer a toothy (ergo frightening) appearance, particularly if he wears such teeth in a collar around his neck. Above all, teeth will scare off demons, who regard these things as reminiscent of their own fangs and horns.

In this vein, it is believed that a wolf's tooth, worn on a chain, prevents nightmares; the wolf will chase the offending mare (or succubus) and sink his lengthy canines into its flesh. Furthermore, the old *Encyclopedia of the Occult Sciences* tells us that "heliotrope which is picked in certain conditions, wrapped in a laurel leaf with a wolf's tooth and carried on the person keeps one protected from slander." Again, the ferocious wolf's tooth will bite or fend off the malice.


## *Color, Shape, and Scent*


Some plant life and certain flowers such as the forget-me-not, for obvious reasons, have amulet qualities, none better than a four-leafed clover, which owing to its rarity and symmetrical shape, is thought to impart rare luck and harmony to life. By the way, even the common and easily found three-leafed clover is useful since it represents the Trinity. But the five-leafed clover (there are such enormities) is absolutely fatal and must be given away upon finding.

Less specific in form, but nonetheless lucky, in the amulet sense, are the natural powers of colors and scents.

Unscientific opinion polls perennially taken have affirmed certain universal affections for certain colors; baby blue, rose pink, and sunny yellow are all-time favorites. Undoubtedly, these choices are based on subconscious word and image associations. The pure hues and pigments alone are secondary to what they presume to represent; after all, baby-blue colored lips, rose-pink eyeballs, and sunny yellow teeth are not great universal favorites despite the polls. It is only when the aforementioned colors are related to such niceties as the sky, spring, and sunlight that their affections hold. As magical "powers"—as trinkets of a generalized form—colors appeal and supposedly function for precisely the same wordplay reasons. Blue is sacred, holy, beneficent, and protective because it has long been called the Virgin's color and invariably is used in Christian iconography related to Mary (Queen of Heaven, or the *sky*).

All shades of red, particularly the richer, deeper hues, are taken as passionate, vivifying colors owing to the obvious blood-sacrifice parallel. Thus, when worn, they are thought effective in arousing passion and inspiration. At the same time, the protective value of red, since it frightens demons who believe it to be part of themselves or tongues of hellish fire, is indispensable when applied to virginal petticoats, crib linings, lips, nails (finger and toes), and face decorations.

Sunny yellow implies optimism, hope, and success—all solar similes have such synonyms; white is purity and protects virginity in a subdued, saintly manner; black imparts solemnity and should be worn when dabbling in sorcery. (Your nefarious activities will thus be blacked out, as it were, from heavenly perusal.) Earth colors stimulate one's earthiness and fertility; silver relates to the moon and mysticism; and according to the occultic encyclopedist, "green has the same powers as the mud baths at Dax . . . !"

Zodiacal color associations appeal to astrological Trinketeers: Gemini favor chestnut (an earth tone); Scorpios, scarlet (passion), and Aquarians, gray—for reasons I cannot explain.

In tandem with this elusive color-power scheme comes the alleged energies of various scents, both fragrant and otherwise. Here again conceptual formations—as opposed to inherent "magic"—are the decisive factors. In addition, olfactory susceptibility is far more prevalent than many think.

With aromas opinions of personal taste play a greater role than in selection of lucky colors, amulets, or talismans. Napoleon, as we know from his love letters, preferred his ladies unbathed, while certain Africans think white men smell like butchered meat. Chanel No. 5 sickens Madame X, bores Madame Y, and thrills the man they both adore. Even so, since ancient times, perfumes, incense, and savory odors have served in thaumaturgic fashion as a form of trinket when worn or suffused in a surrounding. Mohammed regarded fragrance as protective since demons, or jinns, dislike the scent of flowers; Richard Wagner sprinkled himself daily with perfume for musical inspiration, and since Genesis tells us that God enjoyed the "sweet odor" of Noah's sacrifice, religious people have believed pleasant or savory scents put them in favor with the Deity, hence incense in church. The word perfume itself implies the sacrificial function of scent, for the sacrifice was offered through (*par*) the smoke (*fumus*) to the gods.

Natural or earthy fragrances, according to our encyclopedia of the occult, are very propitious, but rather awkward to prepare. Take this formula for something called Friday's Perfume, worn for fertility, amorous, and generally protective purposes (on Friday, the day of Venus). Ingredients: musk, ambergris, aloewood, red roses, all "reduced to a powder, mixed with the blood of doves and the brains of sparrows, made into a paste and then into grains and consecrated with the following words: Deus Abraham, Deus Isaac, Deus Jacob, bless all the creatures of the kinds contained in these odorous grains . . . Per Dominum Nostrum, Amen."

## Security Blankets

The trinkets we have outlined so far are descendants of time-tested ideas and usage. As such they are dear to Trinketeers, who admire nostalgia and tradition. But horseshoes, crosses, and ankhs aside, nothing quite parallels for diversity, variety, and insight the plethora of personalized fetishes, individual idiosyncracies, and self-constructed devices that practically every Trinketeer conceives and cherishes. I call these things "superstitious security blankets" (and in some cases, actual old baby blankets are among the items I mean). Fetishes is perhaps the more Freudian word to employ, but whatever the description, it generally reveals the subtle two-sided nature of superstition (the pro and con) and also helps point up its paper-crutch fallacies.

## The Case of "Chris"

To be specific, I had a friend, named Don, who years ago transformed his car into a veritable fetish on wheels. Imagine an eight-cylinder trinket, baby blue in color, named "Chris" (for Chrysler and St. Christopher), which was believed to be the absolute embodiment of luck and joy. No wonder. "Chris" had been the boon companion of my friend since college days when it was purchased, brand new, with the first hard-earned wages obtained from tending bar in Columbia's famous Lion's Den bistro. At first, no scratch, smudge, or spot was allowed to remain for long on "Chris's" shiny skin, and Don, totally superstitious where his car was concerned, swore to the sky that every time he gave "Chris" a bath, it invariably rained or some Mack truck barreled by and splashed the young coupé with the contents of a muddy puddle. When the inevitable occurred and "Chris" was dented, then scraped, and finally smashed in the rear, Don began to transform misfortune into a kind of "knock-on-wood" benevolence. So long as the car had lost its virginity, so to speak, or had sacrificed its newness to the vagaries of the road, it could be expected to escape worse batterings on the theory "give a little, gain a lot." Interior decorations began to bolster "Chris" against further disaster as talisman and charm were added to fetish in the forms of a St. Christopher medal, a plastic peperon', a chai, and the tassle from Don's high school graduation mortar board (illegally snipped), all dangling from the rear-view mirror. A plastic Madonna with a magnetic pedestal (intended for automotive veneration) adorned the dashboard and to the interior doorframe, a bud vase had been affixed for the presentation of a plastic rose.

The steering wheel and gearshift of "Chris" were candy-striped with blue and white mastic tape and the rear window framed in blue and white pom-pom fringe, carrying out the decorative and protective motif. So adorned and insured, "Chris" served Don as a conveyance to adventure, as a boudoir of love-making, and more importantly, as a castle of pride. When time and built-in obsolescence finally overwhelmed Don's eight-year process of patching (which brought fury to the eyes of the state automobile safety inspector), "Chris" was offered for sale. No one would buy it, not even for scrap, and so Don, who by then had prospered respectably, took a giant step in fetishistic dependence; he arranged for the car to be pressed hydraulically into a six-foot cube and as such it was erected in his garden with the dignity of a Henry Moore sculpture. Of course, prior to its "artistic" transformation, "Chris" was lovingly and ceremoniously stripped of its souvenirs, several of which were transferred to "Linc," the silver and blue Lincoln Continental that Don had subsequently purchased.

### "As It Was"

The famous comedian Ed Wynn was even more persistent than my friend Don, regarding a pair of so-called lucky shoes that he owned for over thirty years, during which time they were soled, resoled, and soled again and patched in every direction. The "Perfect Fool" was convinced that these youthful belongings had brought him success on the stage and he never appeared in that arena without them.

Most everyone of us is inclined toward some form of similar superstitious belief that a particular item, which once seemingly brought us luck, will continue to do so by the magical nature that has somehow permeated its substance. The late operatic tenor, Richard Tucker, obtained Caruso's *Pagliacci* costume for his own debut in that opera in the hopes that some of the great tenor's gift would quite literally rub off on him during the performance. Show business and sports people are fanatical about such things and carry, wear, touch, or possess in some fashion a great myriad of lucky trinkets, mascots, or security blankets prior to performing their thing.

Such dependencies develop in childhood as we begin to associate familiar objects with pleasure and security. Invariably, these are small enough for our tiny hands to grasp and they usually relate to three areas of childhood experience: play, parents, and sleep. The simple rattle or pacifier, which brings security and comfort in times of teething and hunger, loneliness and reprimand is actually the granddaddy of most talismanic trinkets (and the pacifier oddly enough often resembles the ankh). Mother's finger or hair, or some item she perennially wears, like a brooch or pearls, takes on Oedipal dimensions as we grow up and fall back on amulets and habits such as nail biting and hair curling, which may unconsciously remind us of these natural wonderments and reinstate the security and tranquility they represented in our cradle days. (Daddy's necktie or tobacco scent can serve as well.) And when the big world presses from every side and sleep is the only honest escape, we recall with blankets and pillows (and even Teddy bears) and fetal positions those days of safety when we spent most of our lives in a cozy bed.

Harking back to better times (real or imagined) can stimulate all manner of trinketeering ploys and convince the superstitious person that "as it was, so shall it be, if only we can duplicate the details." This emotion, I believe, motivates the periodic waves of nostalgia we seem so prone to employ these days. It's a search for lost youth (i.e., security and comfort), best reinstated in tangible objects such as clothing, styles, hairdos, and physical surroundings.

Passions, especially those of sex, are perfect focuses of this inclination. Because I wore a light blue shirt on that marvelous night so long ago, when young love unfolded for me, unburdened by neurotic constraint, then perhaps by wearing the very same shirt, or at least one just like it, I can, tonight in middle age, enjoy that same blissful simplicity and success. In such cases, the blue shirt often takes the place of personal commitment and sincerity.

## Wearing One's Luck

Often in fairy tales and myths, which seem to bespeak so many unconscious desires, a piece of wearing apparel transforms a character either for good or ill: Siegfried's helmet, which altered his appearance and provided clandestine love; the murderous bridal veil offered by Medea; Cinderella's ball gown and conversely her kitchen rags (one lucky, the other miserable). The Trinketeer is impressed by such things and invests great meaning in wearing apparel for magical purposes: lucky shoes, hats, ties, scarves, gloves, even underwear. Each functions semantically in the sympathetic traditions underlying all tangible superstitions. Lucky shoes lead us on paths of success; talismanic hats inspire us with wit or intelligence; gloves with dexterity; underwear with erotic energies.

The problem with such superstitious dependence can be somewhat facetiously told by imagining a man who has a favorite "lucky" jacket, which, invariably brings him, he thinks, good fortune, love, compliments, and general success. He is so convinced of these results, though he doesn't keep score really to test the premise, that for fifteen years he has worn the very same jacket to every important and pivotal meeting or encounter. Now he is up for a major job, one that requires leadership, poise, and sensibility. True to his unconscious formularization (and blinded by it), our hero dons his lucky jacket, despite its tattered, seedy appearance, its sweaty redolence, and eraded elbows and unashamedly marches into the pin-striped presence of the astonished man he hopes will be his future boss.

The fact is that our childish dependencies, like the lucky jacket, often wear thin, get frayed, and therefore no longer serve us in any measurable way. Neither Ed Wynn's rebuilt shoes nor Richard Tucker's operatic costume would have been worth a dime had either of those two performers lacked talent and skill. Naturally, the fact that each man thought, or believed, his trinket was serving him, did, of course, provide some minor prop for the over-all performance. Just how minor can be readily seen if you consider the horrible results that would have ensued if a tone-deaf rock star had donned Caruso's robes and attempted a performance of *Pagliacci*.

There was an actress who owned a fetish that accompanied her everywhere and was always on stage when she performed. It was an Egyptian scarab, or beetle, very popular as a trinket lo these last three thousand years and presumed to be an infallible bringer of good fortune. This one, carved of turquoise, had been given to the actress, she said, by Noël Coward when she first performed years before in one of his plays. Her resultant success at that time she attributed as much to the scarab as to Sir Noël's or her own considerable abilities. On every occasion when the lady forgot or misplaced the item, she invariably fumbled her lines or bumped into the scenery. What more evidence did I need, she asked, of the psychic powers of this turquoise talisman?

On every occasion? I inquired, or on those when you *knew* you had left the scarab behind? In other words, did you suffer loss of memory or clumsy motion when you thought you had the scarab safely tucked in your bra, but later found it had been at home all along?

After a few minutes of probing contemplation, the actress rather honestly admitted that she had indeed lived through such unacknowledged lapses without disaster, proving that her state of mind and not the actual trinket motivated the good or dire results.


## Little Sheba

Sad are those who demean their own abilities for the mysterious workings of fortune. They win success by hard work and dedication, but maintain it on the paper crutch of a trinket "light as air." The urge to do so and the general reliance on tangible superstitions denotes a lack of confidence in those substantial intangibles that inform so much of success: talent, faith, wit, charm, love, intelligence, and self-esteem. Believing these traits too chancy and unreal, having been buffeted and rejected once too often, the superstitious personality transforms them into symbolic objects that can be fondled and perceived: a scarab for talent, Solomon's seal for faith, a blue shirt for love, and a car called "Chris" for self-esteem. Well and good when lightly held, but dangerous if the individual equates loss of a trinket with loss of promise and ability. On a large and tragic scale such idea formations dominated the Hebrew people when they lost their sacred Temple in the sixth century B.C., until the inspired Jeremiah convinced them that God needs no specific precinct for reverence and that faith may be best found in the "inward heart," not in the gilded chambers of a man-made building. The specious interpretation of history referred to in the Introduction of this book, which purports that the spear that punctured Christ on the Cross was, in fact, an evil talisman responsible for Hitler's rise and power, is another feeble but reckless trinketeering attempt to simplify by a return to childish fairy tales the complex, psychotic motivations that spurred Hitler, on the one hand, and lulled his victims, on the other.

A touching, insightful portrayal of someone whose hopes and actions are locked into a tangible form of superstition was dramatized by William Inge in the play *Come Back, Little Sheba*. Lola Delaney, a former beauty queen now gone to fat, has transferred her hopes and dreams of youth and her sense of security onto the person of a mascot, a lucky animal, called "Little Sheba," a fluffy white puppy, who one day upped and disappeared. Lola continues to search for this symbol of her youth and supposed marital happiness, believing that if the mascot would return, she would then be transformed, in her husband's eyes, into a vivacious, desirable woman. Distracted by these illusions, Lola lazily indulges herself, worsening her marital crisis until her husband, an ex-alcoholic, explodes in a drunken rage. "What are you good for?" he screams. "You can't even get up in the morning and cook my breakfast . . . You two-ton old heifer!"

Jolted by this attack and seeing her husband dragged off to the drunk tank, Lola realizes she must forsake her romantic illusions and tidy up her life—and her house. When her husband returns from his drying out, she reveals a dream she had the night before in which she saw her puppy dead and covered with mud. "I don't think Little Sheba's ever coming back . . . ."[4] says Lola with resignation. "I'm not going to call her any more." Then she sets about energetically to fix her husband's breakfast.

CHAPTER 4

## *Bewitched Equals Bothered and Bewildered*

What do powerless, sexually anxious individuals do who nevertheless want love, power, prominence, and a sense of self? Some turn inward and dry up. Others develop psychoneurotic habits, but somehow survive. Some are cured, rehabilitated by their own strengths or by professional help. A few go mad. Many turn to the world of the weird and dangerous, specifically the occult. According to Ed Sanders, Charles Manson, America's psychedelic sweetheart, chose the latter path and "while counting the days at McNeil Island [a federal penitentiary] . . . began studying magic, warlockry, hypnotism, astral projection, Masonic lore, Scientology, ego games, subliminal motivation, music and perhaps Rosicrucianism."[1] In short, he bewitched himself so that he could someday bewitch others, equally adrift, and in the end establish over them a sort of psychedelic power (some have called it psychedelic fascism), replete with far-out sex and all the other ostensible trappings of potency.

I call this particular superstitious tendency—and it often has sinister psychotic overtones—The Conjuror's Ploy. In it, life is viewed as an enemy camp that will only surrender to the wiles and blandishments of a glamorous and powerful sorcerer (magician, warlock, wizard, witch); in other words, a Conjuror who, by knowing and practicing certain dark and allegedly effective spells, may transform the insecurities born of sexual or potency traumas into the heights of power and fame. Often the Conjuror actually comes to believe in his own rare gifts and mantic achievements. Just as often, the phony knows he's a fraud; but he also knows that attraction to his brand of hocus-pocus, even by the most passive follower, is founded in the very same anxieties he has suffered himself. Thus it is that the Conjuror's slave is often a Conjuror *manqué*, who, failing to achieve his own coven or cult, gladly joins another for at least a brush with magic and its reputed sense fulfillments.

Manson and his Satan's Slaves are possibly the worst extreme of this variety (some include Hitler's nazism on this low point of the scale). At the apparently least dangerous end are those high school kids and suburban housewives who find themselves enthralled with casting beneficent spells (always beneficent), establishing "groovy vibes," and possibly holding a nudie Sabbat once in a while, particularly at Halloween. Midway on the scale of dangerous to frivolous is a concentrated group of people who earnestly believe that the superstitions of witchcraft and sorcery, the medieval syndrome, as we might call it, are in no way merely superstitions (that is, delusions about magic) but are, in fact, proven powers, almost scientific verities, which, when properly understood and mastered, provide all that Manson had, all that the schoolgirl seeks, but do so calmly, coolly, and within the law. If the *true* witch, the closet Conjuror, as we might put it, wishes to do away with Sharon Tate and her friends, he or she need but cast a failproof spell from afar. No messy knives or disembowelments are really required. This true-blue Conjuror will consult his secret *grimoires*, or conjuring books, and in the company of like-minded types will send forth vibrations and glowerings of such proportion and force that no opponent could possibly withstand them. Naturally, sexual power is part of the energy field, and it doesn't matter what kind of sex is performed in the witchcraft ideology. Anton La Vey, the lion tamer turned satanic pope, recommends solitary masturbation when conjuring the devil. For their part, Gardnerian witches (i.e., the white-witch cult founded by Gerald Gardner) simply bathe in salt water and romp about sky-clad, or nude, and sexually tumescent in order to prepare for thaumaturgic activity. Homo- or heterosexual antics, in groups, in duos, or alone are the *sine qua non* of the Conjuror's code, required, we are told, for magical stimulation so that the body and soul may be elevated to the very Everest of the occult. It's not sex for sex, we crave—they pretend—it's sex (or drugs, or sadism, or what have you) for the greater glory of Satan or Diana —or Jehovah or Christ!

To put it in less sensationalistic terms, the Conjuror's neurosis is one that is couched in alibis and gaudy robes. He cannot enjoy sex, of whatever variety, for its own sake, as a purely romantic or orgasmic act. For him, all such sensuous activities must be "elevated" into some ritual form. That is the only way the Conjuror can face the basic sexual disturbances that he has been unable otherwise to mollify or resolve. This chapter will try to show that the usual practices of witchcraft and related sorceries are, by and large, superstitions evolved by impotent people so that they may simulate power, either within themselves or as applied externally to their neuroses.


## Warlock, Witch, Wicca, or What?

A great deal of unnecessary confusion exists concerning the proper definitions of terms used in witchcraft or sorcery circles. Basically, the word witch (ergo witchcraft) is a medieval anglicization employed by Church and civil authorities to describe all suspicious non-Establishment religious or quasi-religious types. These included unconverted pagans, gnostic heretics, Satanists, eccentrics, and some pious members of the Church thought too pious not to be hiding some nefarious ideology. In English the word "witch" is a corruption of *wiche* or *wicca* (i.e., wizard), the name rural people gave to their midwives, herbalists, and quacks. Other languages employ more telling descriptions: *sorcière* (sorceress) in French; *hexe* (witch) in German; *strega* (magician) in Italian. "Warlock" is a Scottish word implying a devil's apprentice, usually a man— hence its common use as a catchall for male witches.

In any event, the word witch is opprobrious, a historically negative description that may be defined as a person (usually a woman) supposed to employ, or suspected of employing, satanic or wicked rituals for the purposes of casting spells. Modern so-called witches, who protest at the nefarious and diabolic implications thus appended to them, seem blind to the fact that they have imposed upon themselves a title created by their enemies and one historically defined in negative terms. But this is their problem, not ours. Those protesting that they are witches only in so far as they practice pagan or "nature" rituals (derived from Anglo-Saxon pre-Christian cults) should forsake the title witch and assume wicca or Druid as a description. Unfortunately for them, in the process, they would forsake all the good media publicity that the word "witch" invariably elicits in the publicist's mind.

Ironically, even the druidic (wicca) variety today conceive of themselves as Conjurors, whether for diabolic or angelic ends. As a result, the "witch" definition seems as good as any for this type. After all, most antidevil witches whom I have met are full-fledged Dualists, that is, firm believers in satanic power even though they may eschew such power. Therefore, for purposes of this analysis, which is concerned with the psychology of witchcraft and not directly with its philosophy, the word Conjuror is the most useful title we have found, so long as it continues to mean one who believes himself empowered with supernatural gifts for the purpose of magically producing miraculous or wondrous effects, especially in terms of love and status.

### The Would-be Witch

Who, then, is the typical Conjuror? To begin with, modern Conjuror types are apt to come from fairly conservative Christian households (or in some rare cases Orthodox Jewish). The confluence of wondrous ritual, miracle, devil belief, and general religious mystery leads one quite easily from the Communion to the Sabbat, conceptually or in fact. Not only Conjurors per se, but also their followers seem to fit this bill—and we are describing both leader and follower under this heading. But religious upbringing is secondary where the potential Conjuror is concerned. Of first importance is the egocentric sense of self, since Conjurors are often confronted early in life with the notion that they are different from others (usually better), generally because of an emphasis on physical beauty or uncanny intelligence. There frequently follows a sexual factor contributing to the "I-am-different" syndrome. In most cases, maladjustment, including highly developed sexual appetite, makes itself felt early in the Conjuror's life; a sense of power, of dabbling in arcana and mystery, results as the precocious child discovers sexual "secrets" long before puberty or before any such development in his peers. This very power usually ultimately—and ironically—turns to a sense of impotence as the taboos of sex are imposed, and this sense of impotence, coupled with a vivid memory and dependence on the power lately enjoyed, is a combustible formula for potential Conjuror delusions.

Burgeoning offbeat sexual behavior and desires are almost inevitably surrounded by a sense of mystique and singularity in the mind of the conjuring child. Conceits may develop in negatively minded cases that unusual sexual leanings are a "curse" or a form of bewitchment (as the Bible implies) and this, of course, establishes the witchcraft ideology. For if one believes himself the victim of a witch, he must by definition believe in the *power* of a witch—and what is power for a witch may, with effort, soon be power for him, as we will see from a specific case. Exclusively homosexual witch cults and practices are common in the contemporary scene, catering to an "I-am-different, ergo alienated" attitude endemic as much to witchcraft as to sexual nonconformity. Very often, this attitude is seen in childhood as a plus, as positive proof of the individual's special, possibly magical status. But though it may be viewed in a non-negative way, this "wondrous" attitude just as easily may lead to conjuring assumptions under the rationale: "I have been made different by nature so that I may master nature, an act which is also different and allowed only to special people." The childish comfort derived from fantasies about special status perfectly complements potential conjuring ideas. In many cases, the small comforts snatched from such fantasies are then enlarged as the sense of loss (impotency) confusingly stimulates the converse sense of singularity (potency) and begins encouraging a formation of life style and philosophy that applies itself specifically to "empowering" (therefore satisfying) the downtrodden individual. What with the inescapable emphasis these days on television, in films, and in paperback books on the general subject of the occult—particularly witchcraft—the choice of conjuring as a positive life style seems almost inevitable in many such cases. Imagine the effect of the following information on a sensitive, sexually confused, and generally isolated preteen or adolescent.

"The power is there, in all of us, and needs only to be pulled to the surface. Energy can be turned toward good or evil and here are the secrets of 'how-to-do-it' witchcraft, including:

"The power of words and spells, voodoo charms, locks of hair, candles, bells, flowers, lotions and potions. Using psychic energy to attract or repel others . . . Sexual seduction spells, charmed sleep, sensuality-awakening spice rubs, true love tea. How to increase your money through witchcraft. The why and how of orgies. And the always useful unwanted-lover spell.

"Dream what you want to, seduce whom you wish, repel your enemies and exercise power over everyone—These are the ideals of witchcraft . . . some of the world's most ancient and jealously guarded secrets."[2]

This is not the spiel of some snake-oil shaman who looks like W. C. Fields. It is taken from the flyleaf page of a popular paperback published in 1971 and entitled, appropriately, *Power Through Witchcraft* by Louise Huebner, who is described as "the world-famous, universally recognized witch"—also known as the official witch of Los Angeles County because she once staged a love spell in the Hollywood Bowl. Yet how intriguing are Ms. Huebner's words for the poor pimply fifteen-year-old who would dearly love to cast spells, seduce others, and be sexually awakened to spice rubs. What is offered to this eager soul is a rather flashy mantic massage parlor for the impotent between the covers of a paperback. I hasten to assure the reader that Ms. Huebner's "ancient and jealously guarded secrets" are a pastiche of simplistic superstitious advice, quasi-historical (true-love tea cake ingredients are "Bisquick muffin mix, Italian sweet sausage . . ."), quasi-pop psychology ("It doesn't matter if you're tall, short, fat, skinny or bald; it is what you project, what you are offering that is important, not how you look"), and mostly a sop to the modern scourge of quiet desperation ("A witch is not an ugly old hag. A witch is a winner . . .").

## Can It Hurt?

Many persons favorable to easy solutions and addicted to the "can it hurt?" philosophy so prevalent these days, may see in such books—and this is just one out of hundreds, including those specifically written for gay, black, male, and kiddie witches—a sort of Dale Carnegie effect: "If it gives a person more self-confidence, more élan, what harm can there be?"

I could jump back to Mr. Manson brooding in his prison cell on the blandishments of "warlockry . . . ego games," and the like, but that might not seem a fair maneuver, although Manson certainly fits in well with the Conjuror type so far described (he was unlovingly raised by a religious aunt, for one thing). But I would rather refer to a dialogue that ensued between me and a young man from Algeria who believed himself bewitched by a Huebner-type Conjuror and had sent a printed plea to a wide number of "witchcraft practitioners, occult scientists (me included!), the New York *Times*, and others" on behalf of his agony.

Sorcery, he believed, was being "used" against him. For the last three years it had taken the form of dreams, "which are not natural," all kinds of noises in the stomach, such as telephone bells, musical instruments, and the like, good and bad odors offending his nose, and optical illusions bemusing his eye. Sleep was tortured, strange feelings in the head and chest were followed by severe pain and assaults from recognizable and unrecognizable voices. Above all, the gentleman labored under telepathic readings of his thoughts, for which he was being punished by the adverse symptoms he had related. This is almost a "desperate" plea, he wrote, from one who was "shocked" that such things could happen in a democracy.[3]

What struck me at once about this case was the sincerity and meaningful despair of the writer, despite his delusions. The other most striking fact about the contents of his appeal was its conformity to the classic symptoms not of bewitchment—as the sender believed—but to the effects of simple or incipient schizophrenia, to wit: hallucination (olfactory, auditory, and visual), persecution mania, thought inconsistency, and the acute sense of outraged helplessness apparent between almost every line.

I contacted this individual and found that he was about thirty-five years old, an Algerian government employee, unmarried, and a recent convert from Islam to Christianity. Of course, the victim was obsessed with the efficacy of witchcraft and would not tolerate any opinion that demeaned the powers of sorcery or suggested a psychoneurotic basis for his malaise. Though he had been to a medical doctor, who found no degenerative organic problem, he spurned the idea of psychiatric help—the invariable reaction and specific problem in most such cases.

Subsequent personal contact with the subject revealed that he suffered from repressed homosexual fantasies. He could, however, see no relationship between his sexual insecurities and the problem at hand, though he was inclined to blame his more scandalous acts squarely on sorcery, not on himself. Further exhortations for psychiatric care went unheeded. A year later, however, I learned that a "breakthrough" had occurred, but what a sorry one. Almost true to form, the victim had decided to become a victimizer and was now engaged in perfecting his own conjuring powers so that he could thwart "by fire" the unnamed antagonists who had bewitched his life.

Here was another mind surrendered to rabid superstition. Eventually, the poor fellow lost his job, not because he avowed witchcraft, as he claimed, but because he was unable, after a time, what with bells in his stomach and the odor of putrefaction in his nose, to conduct his daily routine properly. This example demonstrates precisely how the Conjuror's way, instead of leading to self-assurance and strength (as some believe it does), may actually degenerate into a form of schizophrenia simply because it obscures disease by calling it bewitchment.

## The Case of Margaret-Maggie

Another personal experience afforded me more positive insight in this area, as well as further demonstration of the Conjuror's psychological mechanism. This case concerned a woman well past fifty, who enrolled a few years ago in my course on the occult at New York University. Even at first glance I suspected acute problems of psychoneurosis, possibly psychosis, since the lady wore two ill-fitting sweaters over a heavy dress and appeared to be wearing still another skirt beneath the one I could see. Multiple layers of clothing often bespeak a dangerous level of insecurity and physical, possibly sexual, guilt. In addition, the lady's agitated eyes told of manifold troubles and grief. For several lectures Margaret—as I will call her—sat unmoving in the first row right in front of my desk. She never took notes or asked questions—or answered any. One evening, when the class was leaving, Margaret approached me and softly asked if I were "an ESP." I eventually gathered that she was seeking a sort of witch doctor for help and counteraction since she believed herself possessed by the ghost of a "witch child" who had lived on her street and who had recently died.

In talking with Margaret over the next few weeks, I learned that she came from a Sicilian family that accepted sorcery as a way of life and regarded every craggy old crone—or imperfect child—as a *maga* or *strega*. Her own bewitchment she thought had been instilled by a twelve-year-old spastic who possessed *malocchio*, the evil eye, and who periodically hexed Margaret whenever they met in the course of neighborly visits.

Margaret's real demon was a husband who "beat me on almost every night for the twenty years we were married"; an apparent schizoid, he could not remember his nocturnal attacks the very morning after they had happened. Tyrannized and powerless, yet adhering to her husband in deference to her religion and to her children, Margaret fell back on a childhood fantasy that seemed easily to explain her "curse," to wit: *malocchio* on the part of an "unnatural" *strega* child. For several years this equation sufficed while the poor woman's life deepened in despair and confusion. Nor was the curse released when her husband died in a mental institution, since she never associated her "bewitchment" with him at all. In fact, she believed that he was merely a symptom of the sorcery and not in any way the cause. Even the death of the alleged Conjuror—the child—was not significant since this supposedly evil spirit merely entered Margaret's own person and continued her diabolic machinations from within.

Margaret firmly believed in Satan's power, in witchcraft, and the validity of a curse. She had been chosen for misery, she thought, because early in her marriage, tragically afraid and alienated by her brutal mate, she had briefly found affection in a neighbor's arms. As it turned out, the lover lived in the same building as the spastic child, who was born after the illicit affair and thus seemed to be a later-day punisher for the sexual sin.

As with the hallucinating Algerian, I urged psychiatric care and recommended a clinic near Margaret's home. She was skeptical of such cures and first wanted "an ESP"—another Conjuror—to allay her agonies through sorcery itself. She believed I was such a person simply because I was teaching a course about (but not *in*) the occult. Taking advantage of this confidence, I asked Margaret if her witch-child possessor had a name. She said it had none. "Why not call it Maggie," I asked. "But that's another name for Margaret," she protested. "Exactly," I said, "and this witch child is simply another form of you yourself; the punishing form."

I went on to explain how it was possible for persons who believed in sorcery actually to separate a part of their own personalities and give it an independent life. Margaret's marital enslavement had led her unconsciously to think that an even greater power than her husband was responsible for her hallucinations, pains, insecurities, and confusion—in fact, for all the symptoms "Maggie" provoked (including the fear of punishing cold that resulted in her double layer of clothing).

Throughout, Margaret's conjuring inclination was totally passive. She herself never invoked sorcery except in seeking out "an ESP." She was a Conjuror nevertheless, at least in philosophy, since she took comfort from her troubles and beatings in a belief that some magical, inexplicable force was in fact responsible for life's disorders.

Happily, Margaret eventually came to recognize the "Maggie" effect, especially when she recalled that her own husband was ignorant of his brutalities once he had "slept them off." She saw that it was possible indeed for someone to act against himself, and others, without consciously knowing it. Seeking psychiatric help, Margaret was rehabilitated after a year or so and the witch-child "Maggie" was finally laid to rest.

### Call Me "Scintilla"

Not all Conjuror types are so passive; in fact the opposite is usually true. Carrying through our description of the typical witch, we come to the "glamorous," sexy, power-crazed individual who is never going to allow anyone to conjure her adversely, no matter how strong the sorcery. Rather, she will be the magic superstar conquering everyone and everything she chooses to "spook." Since the person usually involved in such fantasies is a full-lipped, bosomy femme fatale, I believe it more realistic to use the feminine pronoun with this description and to present our type around a lady I will call Joan. Of course, Joan prefers the name "Scintilla," her official coven sobriquet. But since we are attempting to find the real personality beneath the pointed hat, we should stick with the name her parents bestowed on her some twenty-five years ago.

From the first, Joanie was a sex bomb, especially in high school where she made out quite well with the football team, and on occasion with its coach. After barely finishing school owing to her low grades Joanie took a job at a local Woolworth's selling cosmetics. She adored lipsticks, face creams, and sweet-smelling perfumes.

Tight-fitting sweaters were another fondness. She wore them not only to attract masculine attention but above all in the hope that she, like Lana Turner, would be discovered behind a counter and established in a glamorous movie career.

Joanie's reputation in the small town where she lived grew more unsavory every week as news of her dalliances with so-called respectable married men became common gossip. At nineteen, she was branded a full-fledged scarlet woman and femme fatale. Such slander could not be kept from Joanie's parents, who sank in misery and shame at what they soon perceived to be the truth. "She was cursed from birth with a pretty face," her mother lamented. Further scandals and family strife soon put an end to Joanie's natural complacency. She too began to suffer heavy guilt and doubt concerning her seductiveness and vaunted charms. The sudden death of her mother, which the townsfolk in their generosity blamed on the daughter's "way of life," capped her anxiety. Joan became seclusive and penitent. At the same time, her natural "powers" fled, leaving her without identity, uniqueness, *or* fulfillment.

At this point two things could have happened: the young woman might have sunk into an antipathetic way of life in order, subconsciously, to counterbalance her former exuberance. She would then have become a sort of Lola Delaney, the former beauty queen in *Come Back, Little Sheba,* referred to at the end of the last chapter, a dumpy has-been, wallowing in purple dreams. Or, Joan might have honestly found herself, probably with professional help, and thus come to recognize that her natural endowments and sensuality were merely part of her general nature, which, if handled maturely and with taste, could lead to a rich and satisfying married life. For this, however, she would have had to reject the burden of guilt for her mother's death.

Unfortunately, her abnormally strict upbringing and naïveté would not easily allow such liberties. Instead, Joanie turned in a third, more erratic, direction. At Woolworth's she was surrounded by a sea of occultic paperbacks of the type earlier described. Reading through them (she was motivated to do so when she learned that nearly every movie star worth the name was dabbling in witchcraft, astrology, or some such psychic diversion), Joanie discovered that her ample allurements were obviously of a supernatural origin. *Of course* she was unique and that is precisely why everyone hated her and picked on her. Perhaps she *had* caused her mother's death, but not in the ordinary, dreary way. Occultic vibrations, which had flowed from her astral body in protection of her innate mantic potential, were the true offending powers—but powers nonetheless, and, in the long run, redeemable powers at that.

Tentatively, the unhappy girl began experimenting with the candles, incense, and love brews recommended in her Conjuror's guide (at ninety-five cents, a bargain!). Impotency, that sense of loss she had known for months, soon disappeared and what seemed to be a miraculous glow of strength, a new field of power, boldly took its place. Joanie became "Scintilla" and sought out others who proffered the secret Conjuror's truth, the superior sensitivities, all those psychic vibes and lusty emanations she had read about. Steeped in the superstitions of witchcraft, adorned in the appropriate silver chains, black cape, and far-out make-up, Joanie, by the age of twenty-three, was a full-fledged psychic freak—a sort of lady clown, who blindly believed her role in the world was that of a specially endowed and gifted goddess. Whenever she appeared at parties and did her "readings" or cast spells or stripped nude for an "encounter séance," Joanie alibied her indignities with the Conjuror's ploy: "I am special, I'm different. I'm wonderful and full of powerful vibes." Whether potty from too much marijuana or booze, whether being sexually abused or ridiculed, "Scintilla" could feel justified, though debased, for witchcraft tells us "Do as thou wilt"— be yourself (*if* you know yourself); scintillate, even if it means sprinkling your hair with mica dust. Besides, the lady wanted power. Power over slander, over life, over men—and power she finally had.

I knew one individual, rather older than Joan, an avowed witch, publicized in the press as such, a very pretty woman with a history of marital woe and scandal, who in her sixties became a kind of doty old Columbine in cape and silver shoes, good for a laugh on Halloween. The other 364 days of the year, however, Columbine spent her "powers" on bitter tears and loneliness.


### Astride the Broom


The specific superstitions that attract potential Conjurors are those related to historical witchcraft and pagan practices, particularly those of northern Europe during the early Christian period.

Famous classical witches, like the one from Endor in the Bible, or Circe, who transformed men into beasts, or Hecate, the witch goddess of Greece, or even the cunning Medea are not so connotative of the witches we all know—and love—as is the image of a broomborne lady, often craggy, a black cat perched on her shoulder her cloak flying out behind; the sinister female babbling gibberish and hideous formulas like the trio in *Macbeth*. In brief, she is Rosina Dainty-lips, the prototype witch who appears with such memorable gusto in the operatic version of *Hansel and Gretel*. Gruesome, broom-borne, and archly mischievous, especially where children are concerned, Rosina may appear, especially to occultists, the least likely witch and the one, in fact, that has poisoned the public imagination about the *true* nature and description of the hexing breed. Oddly enough, the *Hansel and Gretel* caricature, (and the one in *Snow White*) despite these criticisms, has a basis in reality, at least as pertains to those doty ladies of the Middle Ages who superstitiously believed themselves wondrously empowered with the ability to levitate (or transvect the air), cast spells, and transform humans into sundry shapes, and generally disport themselves in antisocial or eccentric fashion.

Rosina Dainty-lips can most definitely fly her broom, which she accurately calls her "nag" (witches feared real horses, as earlier mentioned). In this wise, she may join the Witch's Dance, or Sabbat, at midnight on the bald mountain, where no taint of vegetation dares appear. Besides, Rosina has provable hocus-pocus powers. She causes Hansel to fall into a trance, after all, and as to her ability to cause metamorphosis, one need but regard her mound of gingerbread cookies made up of what used to be the local boys and girls (shades of Gilles de Rais, the satanic child abuser of the fifteenth century).

Clearly, Rosina is a typical child of her day, whose superstitious beliefs go back, in part, to north European pagans, usually women, faithful to the moon goddess Diana. In the cosmology of this cult, Diana was the center of the universe, who at night possessed the power of drawing the faithful several feet off the ground by some sort of tidal magnetism (moon equals tides is an idea cherished in occultic superstition). This "night riding," as it was called, was usually accomplished by the vigorous flapping of skirts and much attendant shouting and fervor. Possibly narcotic stimulation in the form of psychedelic roots and mushrooms was also employed even in these early days (twelfth century) of the Diana cult. Margaret Murray, the foremost expert on this phenomenon and the scholar who placed witchcraft in its rightfully anthropologic place, reproduced a so-called "flying ointment" such as the ones used by witches (Satanists, that is) and revealed in universal testimony at witchcraft trials.

"The society of witches," says A. J. Clark, who tested Murray's formulas, "had a very creditable knowledge of the art of poisoning . . . There is no doubt, therefore, about the efficacy of [their] prescriptions and their ability to produce physiological effects."[4] A sensation of flying was likely such an effect, especially when we learn that aconite and belladonna—natural hallucinogens—were employed in the ointments witches rubbed between their thighs. From this and other firsthand evidence of actual witches in delirium, women who believed themselves "on a trip" while still in the judge's chambers, it can be seen that flying, whether on broomsticks or on the zephyrs per se, was more than a poetic or eccentric dream. Like most superstitions, it was based on a form of reality improperly perceived by the unsophisticated witnesses (reminiscent of the Druids who thought lightning emanated upward *from* the tree during a storm).

Similar psychedelic stimulation, the knowledge of rudimentary hypnosis, and the efficacy of autosuggestion may have further convinced advocates and leaders of the Craft of their magical abilities, particularly when it came to the other shibboleths of witchcraft such as metamorphosis, invisibility, and trance casting, fantasies universally associated with hallucination.

The Sabbat, which some historians believe to be a mere fiction of the persecuting Church, is too much like well-known rustic ceremonies, the Maypole dance, for instance, to have been pure fantasy either in orthodox or heretical minds. More like an open-air picnic than any lurid present-day ritual, the Sabbat, according to Murray, seemed to have been convened for the most purely congregational purposes, i.e., prayer, marriages, general conviviality, and for the ostensible veneration of fertility forces in nature. In this vein, the devil was considered a "natural" force, identified with the Roman earth god, Saturn, hence saturnalias, which were, in effect, south European Sabbats.

## Superstition Via Sex

The sexual side of historical witchcraft (and fertility rite, then as now, was simply a euphemistic phrase) emerged as the chief attraction of the cult for millions of misused and repressed women, both rich and poor, of the early Christian age. Quite literally kept "barefoot and pregnant," these creatures had no hope of even passing sensuality and lived in a sort of pre-Victorian oppression superimposed with the bugaboos of the medieval Church. Jules Michelet, the nineteenth-century chronicler of medieval superstition, wrote warmly of the sexual motivation behind witchcraft, and thus behind superstition, as he described the restless, sensitive woman of the Middle Ages, so perennially regarded by husband and confessor as a form of the corrupted Eve that "she came to believe herself unclean . . . blushed to love and give happiness to men. Woman . . . she of all others was fain to ask pardon almost for existing at all, for living and fulfilling the conditions of life. A submissive martyr to false modesty, she was for ever torturing herself, actually endeavouring to conceal, abolish, and annul the adorable sign of her womanhood . . . the belly of her pregnancy . . ."[5]

Such women, says Michelet, were bound to concede, once they heard the message that "the Devil only, woman's ally of old . . . in the garden; and the Witch [only they], ever thought of unhappy womanhood, ever dared to tread custom underfoot and care for her health in spite of her own prejudices. The poor creature held herself in such lowly estimation. She could only draw back blushing shyly, and refuse to speak. But the Sorceress, adroit and cunning, guessed her secrets and penetrated her inmost being."[6]

Actual penetration of the "liberated" medieval woman was to occur with some elaboration of the Sabbats where phallic ceremonies, older than Greece, were reinstated as the focus of cult activity, thus establishing the superstitious fallacies of witchcraft by relating them to the realities of sex. By means of an artificial penis, often quite large in size according to the witches' own testimony, great numbers of eager girls and matrons (more so the matrons) could be satisfied, no matter how roughly, by the selfsame "devil." The witch cult, then as now, was a male-dominated activity and the "devil" very often a fallen priest or aristocrat. Properly masked in an animal's head, traditionally a goat's, this devil would probably copulate with the younger and prettier initiates without benefit of artifice. Having spent himself two or three (four or five!) times in the usual fashion, this great goat was then obliged to resort to the artificial device, becoming a Priapus *al fresco*, but one nonetheless quite fulfilling and victorious. Even the Victorian "reverend," Montague Summers, who tended to believe the most egregious superstitions, conceded the use "upon occasion of an artificial penis." Perhaps this dildo *medievalis* was taken to be a broomstick by unsophisticated eyes, and thus "flying" on the broom became not only symbolic of, but also, centrific to the cult.

## Familiar Spirits

The cat, usually black, and sometimes even dogs and birds, played a predictably sexual role in superstitious imagination concerning witches. All such creatures were thought to be familiar spirits, or household demons, who assumed their bestial forms in order to avoid detection while in service to their ladies. The cat as a sexual god (or goddess) was venerated in Egypt as Bast, or Bubastis, but became a succubus, or female sex demon, in Christian demonology. Dogs, because of their shameless and public fornicatory antics, were equally looked upon as debauched. The coincidental fact that elderly and lonely women began, in the fourteenth and fifteenth centuries, keeping dogs, cats, birds, and even mice as houshold pets, led the superstitious imagination, with its predilection for dualism, to assume the worst. The English witch-hunter of this period, Matthew Hopkins, elicited the information from his benighted victims that they kept imps in the forms of poodles, rabbits, and odd-looking hybrids, with names like Pyewackett and Vinegar Tom. Since Hopkins' time, offbeat animals have been universally associated with witchcraft and witches, and the black cat is believed to be the most diabolic and ultimately satanic of them all. If such a cat crosses your path, you may assume it is a witch or her familiar attempting to destroy the sanctity of your journey (and future) by treading through the sacred symbol, the cross, made by your shadow.

Other sexual and sinister ideas (often in the medieval mind, the two were identical) were and still are associated with witches or

Conjurors. The sinister notions, of course, originate in the fantasy idea that witches had special psychic or magical powers. This delusion was (and is) the result of the publicity created by the confluence of Church hysteria and witchy arrogance. But the sexual antics of these people then and now are far less fantastic in origin or practice. After all, Michelet's repressed and tyrannized housewife still haunts the manicured world of suburbia in the 1970s, or appears fitfully in classrooms or symposia devoted to the occult, hoping for a chance to express herself in the most basic and "magical" way ever conceived. Every believer in witchcraft knows this fact, possibly even respects the need. Sexual tension is historically fundamental to the Conjuror's ideology. When cloaked in superstitious conceits, couched in terms of psychic vibrations, love brews, auras, and familiars, the erotica of witchcraft, may become acceptable even to the most inhibited and frigid amateurs. Once accepted, a certain sense of fulfillment, even joy may be experienced.

## Whither Witchcraft?

Medieval witchcraft, the cult of women, was according to Pennethorne Hughes, "a religion at all events in promise of joy."[7] If joyful, what then can be wrong with it? Why does the Conjuror's superstitious activity, in the past and today, imply neurotic or possibly dangerous tangents, if indeed it is sexually fulfilling and a "religion of joy"? Is a debunking of witchcraft simply a mask for the age-old sport of witch-hunting? Is it a cloak for uptight outrage, or a sanctimonious masquerade?

Witch-hunting, especially by religious crusaders, is totally outdated and unnecessary. But laissez-faire is equally unwise. What should concern us about witchcraft today are questions of mental health and human dignity. Any critical investigation of the so-called Craft and its advocates must be governed by these concerns. When viewed as a problem of psychology, the Conjuror's ploy will eventually be seen as a rather cruel exploitation of sexual anxiety and the superstitious attitudes born of such anxiety.

Every potential Conjuror, active or passive, every would-be witch, as she lights her candles or brews her potions, should ask herself (or himself): "Is this the only way, the honest way, by which I can find love or strength or status. Is this 'love' I seek really love, or merely an outlet for my frustrations. Is it power I want or simply revenge; revenge against those who have repressed me and mocked me and caused me grief? When the incantation is over and my beloved appears at my bed, will I be able to respond honestly, be a warm and loving *individual* or a paperback imitation with a personality imposed on me by a sharpie who couldn't care less about my happiness or personal success? In a word: am I responsible for *me*—or am I just a pawn in some phony magical master plan?"

## *The Evil Eye*

Mention has been made of the evil eye, an idea apparently older than civilization and rooted in the appeasing tradition discussed in Chapter 1. For Conjurors, affectations about "burning, all-knowing" eyes are stock in trade. To the uninitiated, nature seems to have marked the psychic, conjuring individual with compelling eyes, and as a result, *malocchio*, the evil look, is a favorite superstition in many cultures. Even cats are presumed capable of this ocular magic, particularly witch's cats.

Taken to its extreme, such *malocchio* can reduce an enemy to ashes (Conjurors are partial to the nonsense of spontaneous combustion); in its mildest form, the evil eye will cause others to submit to your will—a process known as fascination in the Middle Ages—making them sexually submissive, or dominant, depending on your particular desires.

Perhaps the most telling information about the true nature of the evil eye was related by Edgar Allan Poe in his story *The Tell-Tale Heart*. Here, a psychotic individual murders an innocent old man not actually because of an *evil* eye, but because of a sickly one "all a dull blue, with a hideous veil over it . . . ." It is the murderer himself, power-crazed and hallucinatory, who concocts the evil nature in his victim's eye. Others would see it for what it was, a defective organ, more a burden to the old man than a means of "fascination." To put it another way: *honi soit qui mal y pense.* If you see someone glaring you down with an "evil eye" make sure it is not your own eye that in perceiving is evil and superstitiously defective.

Fear of being cursed or hexed underlies general anxieties about the evil eye and all other aspects of witchcraft today as in the past. So intense was this fear that the burning courts of the Middle Ages sat beneath huge protective crucifixes when questioning alleged witches. Such remnants of the superstitious past may still be seen in French and Italian courtrooms, among others. The ability to cast spells, whether white (benign) or black (malicious), is taken as a definitive sign of all self-proclaimed witches and is, in fact, one of their most effective deceptions, founded as it is on the universal idea that specific concentration by "gifted" persons can produce peculiar results.

Colin Wilson, who distinguished himself in England as an "angry young man" in the 1950s, has turned to occultic advocacy in recent days. According to his own accounts, Wilson thinks he may have exercised the evil eye on a querulous old neighbor who died of a heart attack soon after Colin wished him dead.[8] Writing in the New York *Times*, on the Op-ed page of all places, Wilson also declared his belief in the hexing powers of natural (that is unpublicized) witches. One had put a spell on a friend of his and sure enough "he had terrible luck for months—dreadful things kept happening to him."[9] Wilson sees this as a power to do harm by "ill wishing." Later, in Chapter 9, we will discuss the actual power of coincidence as it functions in the superstitious mind; our aim for now is to expose the business of hexing, whether in the simplistic though civilized forms Colin Wilson accepts ("if thoughts could kill" and so forth) to the more elaborate and fearsome voodoo practices of sticking pins in a doll.

### Voodoo Practices

A full description of voodoo and related Afro-Caribbean sorcery is beyond the purpose of this book. Suffice it to say that voodoo practices—and the witches of Europe engaged in their own versions—are highly dependent on the power of suggestion and on a form of psychedelic fascism already explained. Worked into a frenzy by dancing and possibly narcotics, Haitian practitioners of voodoo eventually lose themselves in a sort of delirium which enables a select few to become the *chevaux*, or horses, for the *loa*, or gods, of the region who supposedly can possess the unsouled individual. The over-all antics are supervised by a priest and priestess responsible for initiating "punishing" rituals, including the well-known sticking pins into a doll. Fifth faths are the names of such surrogates in Gardnerian or Celtic witchcraft, but essentially they are the same: a poppet or rag doll is constructed in either male or female form and to it is appended some personal item of the individual chosen to be cursed. This indispensable item may be a swatch of clothing, a lock of hair, or nail parings (superstitious people fear losing the last two bodily items because of potential voodoo hexing). Affixed to the doll, the personal factor somehow transforms rag and string into a substitute presentation of the living person. Pins stuck in "his" heart or spleen, or other indignities performed à la sorcery, will therefore cause a sympathetic reaction to take place in the real being. Possibly he may have a heart attack, like Colin Wilson's "victim," or merely a "stabbing" pain in the chest.

The operative factor in all such hexings is the concomitant knowledge of the victim regarding his curse. In Haiti, he will often find the dreaded pin-cushion doll on his pillow or astride his threshold. Autosuggestion and self-fulfilling prophecy now take over as the seeds of superstition (the cursing) find fertile soil in the frightened mind. Persons indifferent to such things or unknowledgeable of the punishment will conduct their daily routines with the usual ups and downs—unless they believe they have been cursed even without any tangible evidence.

## Metamorphosis

Not all spells are destructive, as noted earlier in relaying the nostrums of the Los Angeles witch, Ms. Huebner. Many modern Conjurors, in fact, insist that they are in business only to issue beneficent charms. But the implication is always that evil powers are fully within their grasp and, when angered, could be expended. A warlock I once confronted on a television talk show boasted so greatly of his magical powers that I challenged him to transform me then and there into a toad. "You're already a jackass," he countered. When I insisted, despite his barbs, Mr. Warlock finally snapped that turning men into toads was distinctly malicious, in the category of black magic, and though he could do so easily, he preferred more productive activities.

"Very well," said I, "let me bring you a toad; change it into a man. Surely that might be considered a beneficent gesture." Naturally, even that challenge was left unmet, the point being that the magical power indispensable to the authenticity of any witch, regardless of inclination or generation, was not there, never could be, and never will be without recourse to trickery and dependence on popular gullibility.

## The Social View

Even so, witches and their ilk hunger for recognition and status, ultimately for love, even as anyone else in this complicated world. Their method of coping, however, is to seek instant power via the *grimoire,* or conjuring book. Often they carry off their "act" with such flair and conviction that self-deception becomes a deeply entrenched way of life, and as such appeals to others who also seek status, but who, being less artful, are content to follow and believe. These people cheat themselves by such beliefs because they must fall back on antiquated notions of the universe and on the weaknesses of others, not upon their own inner strengths or potentialities. Naturally, in order to maintain an air of bewitchment, the Conjuror must also manage to support a pose of superiority and godliness. Arthur Lyons, in his incisive book *The Second Coming: Satanism in America,* refers to the "know-it-all" glint in the eye of Conjuror types who believe "they have acquired powers not normally found in outsiders." These glints, of course, are merely masks of "acute feelings of inferiority."[10]

All this may seem a harsh indictment, possibly a condemnation. But, unfortunately, persons of the Conjuror variety need debunking more than most because of the coven concept intrinsic to their calling, the socio-political aspect, one might call it, that tends to develop followings, cults, and possibly movements which eventually may have fascistic and criminal dimensions.

The blinding of horses and dogs in one suburban New Jersey town recently shocked American sensitivities when reported in the media, especially when it was learned that the outrages had been performed as part of satanic rituals (blinded animals are supposed to be able to "see" the demon). Our young people, more so than horses and dogs, are falling victim to the "witchcraft thing." I have seen police files of cases in which teen-agers have engaged in brutal crimes as part of power rituals. In one such instance, a so-called warlock persuaded his followers to drown him so that he might obtain instant power in hell, the glorious fate, he believed, of those who are "done in." The fate of his followers was to go to prison for homicide.

A French ethnologist studying sorcery in Normandy reported in *L'Express* magazine that she believed witchcraft could help people "in a certain way to understand their troubles,"[11] that witchcraft can open doors to personal insight, which might otherwise be locked or sealed. In many minds, Conjuror's fantasies, like any form of adventure, presumably stimulate change and possibly self-confidence. But witchcraft is a very brittle crutch in this regard. The change it may cause can be for the worse, as in the case of "Scintilla," and the self-confidence it seems to create will likely dissipate with the first unanswered ritual. Above all, because witchery caters, as it must, to a neurotic need for sudden power and dominance, it comes to rely on superficial signals and shallow effects. Since one of the most prominent of these effects, implicitly promised by all sorcery, is sexual love, the possibilities for exploitation and abuse of the lonely are always lurking in this area. This equally applies to promises of wealth, health, vindication, and success. Financial bilking may logically result. Worse yet, the insecure and possibly schizoid individual—both leader and follower alike—may be robbed of all chances for professional help and rehabilitation because of his dependency on superstitious myth. Such help is almost invariably needed. In discussing Satanist witches with whom he lived for two years in San Francisco, Edward J. Moody, writing in *Religious Movements in Contemporary America* quite categorically states that among the diverse types of people he met in the Satanist church, "all were deviant or abnormal in some aspect of their social behavior."[12]

With this evaluation in mind, a good formula for those who crave bewitchment, of whatever form, would be to ask themselves if the conjuring powers they seek might not be better and more fully realized in show business or in a massage parlor. In either arena, "stardom," i.e., power, love, sex, and glory, is at least embroidered with obvious, undeceptive tinsel and frippery. In witchcraft and the Conjuror's world, the greasepaint and histrionics, no matter how dehumanizing, are too often taken to be aspects of the divine. And —if neither show biz nor brothel are found to work, the would-be Conjuror is next exhorted to consult a dependable therapist before racing to the pantry in order to expropriate the family broom.

CHAPTER 5

## *Living with the Dead*

A striking photograph in a recent book about myths and anthropology shows an elderly New Guinean gentleman in profile, quite peaceably asleep, his head pillowed upon a well-bleached skull of an ancestor, with whom the sleeper hopes to communicate through dreams. Though grandfather's skull may be a rather uncomfortable pillow, it does provide, symbolically or otherwise, a tangible bond between man and one of his greatest anxieties, indeed the anxiety that may well be fundamental to the formation of all superstitious ideas and beliefs. The thing is death, that old "lean fellow that beats all conquerors," according to Thomas Dekker; the inevitable enigma that shall have its day no matter what we say or do.

And with death and dying there comes another anomaly, possibly an even more enigmatic consideration than death itself and that is the product of death: the dead—us, we who are now walking about quite lively and sentient, who will, according at least to empirical evidence (and biblical ideology), be turned to dust and nothingness. The Preacher of Ecclesiates (9:5) puts it this way: "the dead know not anything," they do nothing, they are nothing.

Nothing? Contradictory evidence may also be found in the Bible, which speaks of spirits, ghosts, and immortal souls. From ancient Egypt to the current craze for reincarnation, the idea persists: man may ultimately die, but he need not stay dead. And if he only appears dead but actually lives on in some altered form, still conscious, still knowing, and still capable of action—while fearless of death—if this is true, then a dead man is a formidable thing, one worthy of as much superstitious or propitiatory concern as is death itself.

Is this why the sleeper from New Guinea keeps contact with the skull? Is it to stimulate memories of the past, to show respect, to forestall forgetfulness of him who has departed, to protect the sleeper from the inevitable, to remind him of his *own* mortality? All these motivations are indeed present in his morbid choice of pillow. They are present in each of us when confronted by the death of others, whether we are philosophical and sober (even so we will memorialize the departed) or whether we are emotional and confused. In some cases, our attitudes about death and the departed may border on superstitious and irrational explanations which may be nevertheless considered perfectly normal and restorative. People dreaming about a recently deceased relative or friend who convincingly perceive that individual whole and happy and hear him say: "I am at peace," derive a modicum of beneficial self-help from their dream despite its more obvious psychological explanations.

Religious ceremonies, the funeral itself, and activities related to mourning, though often rooted in ancient superstitious origins have transitory value in affording courage, direction, and relief. Consider the prayer for the dead, the Kaddish, in Judaism, which calls upon the bereaved to stand up with others, grief-stricken like himself, and affirm his faith in God despite bereavement. This affirmation per se may be strengthening and comforting. But of even greater value, it seems to me, is the community nature of the prayer; the sharing of grief.

This company that misery seeks is not for purposes of morbid perversion; it is for unity in confusion, for confraternity in the face of what Camus called "the absurdity" of death. As such it should be encouraged and it explains the persistence of funeral obsequies: the wake, the visits, the special considerations and symbols of mourning. These are the vital reactions that support the living despite their alleged functions on behalf of the dead. They affirm life itself by contrasting, no matter how brutally, the marvel of our own animation with the passivity of *rigor mortis*.

## *The "Dear Departed"*

But there is an aspect of death, and those who die, that weighs heavily in superstitious terms and often leads to incapacitating guilt and fear and thus to a plethora of useless activities which may evolve into a form of living death. This problem is rooted from time immemorial in the belief in ghosts and the dread of all things moribund in terms of punishment and revenge. It creates, in extreme cases, a panic of expiation in the survivor, who feels himself spied upon by vengeful, ghostly eyes, who covers himself, not so much in mourning as in guilt, and who seeks to create a continual barricade against the "dear departed," whom he regards as neither dear nor, in fact, departed at all. Such people, saddened and afraid, who construct superstitious antidotes against the vengeful dead may be called Expiators. Their reactions range from draping mirrors and doors with crepe to attending hopeful sessions at the spiritualist's table seeking a final word of forgiveness from the terrible wrath of the spirit who has "passed over." Often, in fact, this spirit remains within the Expiator himself, for it enlivens in him a secret craving to live a form of existent death while in the throes of persistent punishment.

Knowledge of the mechanism of guilt feelings in psychology is essential to the understanding of the Expiator's actions and beliefs. According to psychoanalysts, guilt, as opposed to shame, arises out of the conflict between those values learned in childhood and basic primitive instincts repressed in the unconscious. The well-known battle between the Ego and the Id may be cited in this situation, in which impulses of the Id constantly bombard the Ego until it is weakened and overthrown with all its childhood values (the aggregate of which is sometimes called the Superego). In some cases, the individual (the Ego) develops guilt feelings without necessarily submitting to primitive instincts. His unfulfilled wish to vent such feelings is enough to establish the unconscious disapproval syndrome, including depression, bitterness, and bouts of irrationality. Of course, only someone with a fairly well-developed sense of values (whether acted upon or merely inculcated) can experience the violation of those values, on the one hand, and the guilt that subsequently occurs, on the other. A man unacquainted with and unmoved by the biblical commandment "Thou shalt honor thy father and thy mother" may unconsciously or even consciously wish his parents dead without suffering a guilty ego.

Because most people develop values of the Superego in childhood, guilt resulting from violation of such values is often related to parents and family. The death of kin is therefore a common trigger for the full-blown onslaught of guilty neurosis and its attendant affects. There is such a thing, of course, as normal, or justified, guilt. But as Dr. Ross Thalheimer explains: "Where the feeling of guilt is free floating, or where, either quantitatively or otherwise it is considered to be *inappropriately* related to the act in question, a therapist may speak of it as 'neurotic' rather than as 'normal' guilt."[1] It is the inappropriate application that the Expiator, because of a superstitious inclination, subsumes into the general realm of irrational belief.

## The Case of the Garish Vase

The case comes to mind of a young woman, about thirty-five, whose widowed mother was suffering from a terminal illness. The daughter, being single, was left in charge of the parental home while the mother was hospitalized. As mistress of the manse, the young woman began assuming a sense of dominance over her absent mother, who had always been something of a martinet, and accordingly set about rearranging the furniture and wall hangings in accordance with her own tastes, which were ever at variance with those of her parent. In the course of these decorative changes, the daughter "accidently" broke a particularly garish vase revered by the dying woman. After several weeks of playing mistress to her mother's house, the young woman grew bored with the place and allowed it to fall into neglect. Nevertheless, she continually assured her mother in the hospital that all was well at home and exactly as the older woman had left it.

Upon learning of her mother's death, the daughter suddenly panicked without knowing why. Grief alone could not explain her reactions, particularly in light of the rather cool affection she had maintained for her mother since adolescence. Her fears were, in fact, related not so much to her mother's death, which was merely a triggering, but to a superstitious anxiety that the dead woman's ghost would now return to her home—as ghosts reportedly do—discover the changes, *and* the broken vase, and predictably wreak vengeance. In a desperate attempt to forestall this wrath, the daughter hastily draped all the mirrors in her mother's home with sheets in the quaint belief that the dead woman's ghost, not being able to see its own reflection, might believe itself in the wrong house. Indeed, hanging crepe on the door or around the portals of a dead man's home is also intended to disguise the house and thus protect it from haunting.

The denouement of the young woman's story fulfills the extremes of the Expiator's guilt anxiety, for as she was hanging a bedsheet across a particularly large mirror in the dining room, the daughter fell from the ladder, broke her lower leg, and had to be hospitalized. Punishment, symbolically duplicating the broken vase, had now joined guilt in the usual and painful resolution of such neurotic tendencies.

As will shortly be seen, most venerable death rituals, or superstitions, tend to reinforce ancient anxieties about the punishing dead. As already stated, when these are regarded as "strategies of solace," such activities may be functional (a few, however, are too egregious to be considered strategies even under the most trying circumstances). But when taken as acts of expiation per se, in imitation of their original formation, then that expiation tends to denote a sense of guilt which may be totally unwarranted and inappropriately related. Each mourner therefore becomes responsible to himself (the ultimate responsibility) in determining just how guilty he ought to feel, if at all, concerning the death of a relative or friend. In some cases, a sense of failure and of unworthiness may indeed be justified; that is for the individual to decide. What is rarely if ever justified is irrational punishment meted out via superstitious rituals. Even the most guilty and hardened criminal is allowed an appeal. For Expiators, the appeal must be to reason; they must know the sources of their guilt, analyze its appropriateness, and then sensibly work out the trauma through rational expiation, such as in therapy or as religion may afford. In addition, they would do well to understand the psychological—as opposed to spiritual—origins of the activities performed in tandem with death. Once stripped of their almost sacred solemnity, many of these ploys may come to seem as inappropriate as unjustified guilt. With such understanding, the individual may protect himself from becoming what William James described as a "sick soul" burdened with chronic anxiety disguised in part as religious or reverent respect for death *and* its attributes.

### Memento Mori

Most universally observed burial and funeral customs originated in prehistoric times. Neanderthal graves, some seventy thousand years old, have been unearthed that indicate ritual burial in which the arms of the corpse are folded and tied and the body set down among ceremoniously arranged shells and pebbles. In the Zagros Mountains of Iran, a sixty-thousand-year-old grave was unearthed in which flowers had been buried with the corpse. During Cro-Magnon times, some fifteen thousand years ago, bodies were tied with leather thongs to inhibit reanimation, painted with red ocher, a symbol of life (lumps of such ocher have been found in European graves), and then surrounded with boulders, primarily to prevent the corpse from rising and haunting the environs. This cautionary act is the origin of tombstones and grave markers, which are monuments, in their own way, to the fears of primitive man, who assumed the dead would rise from their graves because they appeared so lifelike in his dreams so soon after burial. (As noted, such dreams are natural occurrences in bereavement.) Dream figures ill perceived as spectral realities may be the origins of all ghostly conceits and the anxieties born of such "visions" seem to have instigated all sorts of precautions at the grave, where it was presumed the specter resided awaiting its chance to "escape."

## The Egyptian Funeral

No society of the past, or present (except perhaps in America today), parallels ancient Egypt for funerary considerations, most of them rooted in religious or superstitious fears and the need to inhibit reanimation of the dead. The most conspicuous pile of inhibiting boulders still on view is the pyramid of Khufu near Cairo, which was constructed as a Pharaonic tomb. The Egyptians of that period believed perfect preservation of the corpse as a mummy was necessary for its survival in the afterlife (which survival precluded its need to reappear in the "current" life as a ghost). It was not the corpse as such that journeyed "to the West," as the Egyptians referred to their paradise, but rather its double or astral body called the Ka—the first elaborated concept of a soul in recorded history. Unless propitiated with food and other worldly endowments, the Ka might languish and then rise to haunt the living or else bear angry condemnations of his kin to the netherworld, where human deeds were weighed on a scale of justice. This vengeful attitude associated with the dead may be related to a curious Egyptian ideology concerning life that Gaston Maspero, the pre-eminent Egyptologist, describes in his seminal work on the societies of the ancient Middle East. "In Egypt," he writes, "man does not die, but someone or something assassinates him. The murderer often belongs to our world . . . another man, an animal, an inanimate object . . . Often, though, it belongs to the invisible world and only reveals itself by the malignity of its attacks; it is a god, a spirit, the soul of a dead man that has cunningly entered a living person . . . and death speedily ensues . . ."[2]

Thus assassinated, the dead man's Ka awaits its own peculiar fate. Either the corpse will be properly embalmed and revered, entombed with his favorite treasures and household equipment, protected by amulets, talismans, and holy texts, or else he will be dishonored with a poorly preserved mummy, portending for the Ka a "second" death and an eternally burdened heart. In such a case, the embittered Ka may resort to use of a funerary scroll, a book or guide for the dead, which when read enables the mummy to be revived (as a "ghost") and thus return to the world of humans where it may suck the marrow and the blood of guilty kin, just as some wandering spirit had earlier afflicted the man who once it was.


## Mourning Rituals

The notion that death is invariably malignant and unnatural leads directly to the formation of guilt associations in the minds of survivors, for if their own beloved was murdered by some unnatural force, be it a god or a ghost, could it possibly have been as a punishment not only for his sins but also for theirs? Even today, many people, especially bereaved parents, regard their loss as a chastisement for some personal turpitude, some sinful thought or immoral deed. Many so convinced beg forgiveness at the wake or graveside; others offer huge sums of money "in memory" of the dead, but, in fact, it is in aid of expiatory charity for their own misdeeds, real or imagined. Maxim Gorky said: "We all drive each other into the grave . . . First we feel ashamed about it, then frightened by our guilt."[3]

In post-Egyptian times, fear of a vengeful corpse prompted several commonplace activities still in use regarding the dead. Washing the body, a prerequisite in Judaism and Islam, and often in Christianity, is based on the theory that evil spirits abhor water and will thus stay away from the corpse, or, more cogently, be inhibited within the corpse and thus prevent its ghostly animation. Candles burning by the body and coffin function in the same way; they frighten demons and wandering spirits. The use of burning candles at wakes can be seen in Japan among Shinto adherents as well as in Western ceremonies. Light, burning torches, the sun itself, were sought to keep harm from the survivors as they carried the corpse to its final resting place. The funeral procession was in fact an illuminated parade; the word funeral derives from *funus*, which in Latin means torch or taper. Today, automobiles in a funeral procession turn on their headlights in remembrance of the torchlight procession, which now, as in the past, must move unimpeded to the grave site, lest the corpse, like Finnegan at his wake, suddenly decide, maliciously, to revive itself.

Another use of funerary flame is found in the kindling of memorial lights, usually on the anniversary of the death. This indicates to the ever-watchful departed that his kin have not forgotten him and therefore do not deserve his obloquy.

The most elaborate use of fire as protection from and for the corpse, occurs in cremation, which among Hindus and the ancient Greeks was mandatory on the theory that the soul could not otherwise escape the flesh. But the practice dates back to Neolithic times, from which funerary urns housing ashes and human bones have been preserved. Scholars believe burning of corpses was universal in the Roman world, except among the Jews, who feared that intentional destruction of the corpse would interfere with resurrection, an idea clearly adopted from Egyptian beliefs. Christianity carried on this Jewish tradition, and as the new faith spread, the practice of cremation retreated. Orthodox Jews today eschew burning the dead not only because it may impede resurrection (although the Bible refers to the cremation of the ill-fated King Saul in I Sam. 31:12) but because of a quaint belief that relates to Adam and Eve. Since the legendary parents of man hid themselves from God, after eating the fruit, "amongst the trees in the garden" (Gen. 3:8), this was taken as a sign that their descendants, now mortal, should be buried in wooden coffins, (i.e., trees) and therefore never burned.

Though evidence of burying men in dugouts (canoes) exists—and these do resemble the traditional coffin—greater merit can be given to expiatory undercurrents when it comes to the origins of coffins or boxlike burial containers. Primitive bodies were lowered unencumbered into the grave, although, as noted, many of them were either tied or bound and all weighed down with what were hoped were unmovable rocks. As survivors became more alarmed about ghostly animation and as the opportunities for building elaborate pyramids and tombs diminished, men turned to more obvious means of encasement and inhibition, notably the dugout—reversed over the body—and then later, the chest. Indeed, early medieval coffins were precisely chests, bound by chains and locked to keep the dead in their place. A sturdy box could also preserve the corpse for resurrection and thus enable him to lie in peace, unmotivated to punish his survivors who may have improperly buried him or who sinned against him in life. The practice of beheading the corpse, thus rendering him ignorant (ergo inanimate), and of placing the severed head between fettered legs, further indicates a guilty and grisly fear of ghosts. "Rest in peace," as we can see, is only half the sentiment: "And leave *me* in peace" is the unspoken phrase.

Flowers, wreaths, bushes planted on the grave, and beds of ivy may appear today to be decorative and reverent in origin, but they were actually conceived by Expiators to protect themselves from the vengeful dead. The circular wreath over the grave inhibited spirits from entering or exiting since such creatures are believed incapable of breaching a circle (symbol of life and unity). Flowers rich in perfume also inhibit spirits, and plants, especially evergreens, give promise of renewal and resurrection, thus appeasing the corpse and keeping him at bay. Possibly flowers are also substitutes for the food ancients placed in tombs to placate the hungry ghosts and prevent them from invading the household kitchen for a post-mortem snack.


## Passage Beyond


Once the family is convinced that their loved one is properly interred, it follows that religious rituals be pursued to ease the deceased's passage into the afterlife and thus inhibit his restlessness—and vengeance. From Pharaonic Egypt to modern times, prayers for the dead have combined propitiatory, expiatory, and magical formulas. In ancient Ur, a monarch's family (all save his heir) was so intent on assisting easy passage for the dead that they dutifully accompanied him on the fatal journey; fatal for them as well as for the corpse. Mounds uncovered by archaeologists in the Tigris-Euphrates region show hundres of skeletons arranged around the burial chamber of a king. Similar royal burial pits, heaped with skeletons, have been found in northern China dating from the Shang dynasty, around 1500 B.C. The outlawed "Suttee" ritual of India, obliged the devoted widow (*sati*) to join her dead husband on the funeral pyre. In this way she assisted his passage beyond and ensured her own fidelity to his memory. Surely such human sacrifice is the ultimate form of expiation, akin to the modern sentiment heard in mourning: "I want to die with him [or her]; let me also go, let me perish, let me not remain behind!"

Often such extreme emotions are motivated by profound love and sorrow, the intermingling of which can be painful indeed. But in some cases, the remorse of a Hamlet may be evinced. He, discovering Ophelia's funeral and believing himself responsible for her suicide, leaps into her grave and bitterly commands the diggers to throw "millions of acres on us . . ." Most of us, even the most guilt-ridden Expiator, will preferably fall back on prayers of atonement, which are believed useful in assisting the dead and procuring the status: *requiescat in pace*. The Hebrew Kaddish, mentioned earlier, is not precisely a prayer for the dead, but actually a paean in praise of God, and functions more as a "strategy of solace" than in any propitiatory or expiatory way—although Jews believe that a son may bring dishonor to the memory of his dead parents if he does not carry out this duty. In this sense, it is practically universally performed even among indifferent Jews—since they believe it to be expiatory in content. A specific "passage" prayer, to assist the dead in their somber journey, does appear in the Jewish liturgy and is recited at the grave and thereafter so that the deceased may be brought up from Sheol, the nebulous netherworld where spirits wander prior to the peaceful sleep preceding resurrection. This prayer of remembrance (Yizkor) specifically calls for the repose of the deceased, whose name is inserted at the proper place, and includes the phrase "open unto him [or her] the gates of righteousness and light . . . Oh, shelter him or [her] for evermore under the cover of Thy wings . . ."

Catholic ritual in this regard is even more elaborate and often suffices expiatory inclinations by the duties of merit it imposes upon the living. The prayers recited at Catholic ceremonies are bound up with the aforementioned Sheol, or purgatory, which in Catholic doctrine becomes a place of final atonement for venial sins by those dead souls who are not previously damned to hell. Aquinas believed family prayer and merit could help lessen the purgatorial punishment of the soul; hence the appearance of indulgences, commutations of temporal punishment due to sin, which may be in the form of specific charity. The Hindu-Buddhist tradition recognizes a form of purgatory and requires attendant prayers, offered by monks, for the perfection of the karma, or merit, of a departed soul in the hopes that it may be recycled closer to the ultimate goal of paradise (nirvana): a status of nonbeing where the pattern of reincarnation ends. In Islam, paradise is a specific place and so is hell. Prayers for the dead are recited at the mosque and at the grave site, which is a mound heaped up with small boulders. The prayer resembles the Jewish Kaddish. An implication of fear of the dead can be heard in the sentiment that Muslims state at the funeral of a loved one: "Oh God, if he did wrong, then let his offense pass without punishment . . . deprive us not of his reward and try us not after his death."

## Spectral Visitations

The persistence of ghosts in superstitious thought and their formatory influence on burial rituals does not end for the Expiator with the closing of the tomb or the coffin lid. Infused with a dread of haunting, supported by unconscious guilt, the Expiator may seek actual contact with the discarnate spirit in the hopes of atoning for his wrongs in the very presence of the deceased. In superstitious ideology, phantoms are generally unapproachable since they are characteristically overwrought and ill tempered, riven with envy as they see themselves cut off from life, love, and warmth.

The lion's share of frightful apparitions—true to their name—are bent on torturing or killing the living, whether the specter be the Japanese Kohada, a skeleton ghoul immortalized by the artist Hokusai, or the punishing ghosts of Timor Island, described by Frazer, who assiduously seek out those warriors who slew them. These warriors are thus forced to hide away for two months after battle in a special hut that supposedly confuses the ghosts and eventually thwarts their purpose. Modern mourners don black, and women veil their faces, for the very same reason that the Timor warriors hide away, that is to disguise or sequester themselves so that the aggressive spirits will not know precisely who is who among the bereaved. Tearing the clothing and covering the head in ashes further mask the living and make them appear less enviable and punishable in the eyes of the embittered and vengeful dead.

In an extremely penitent mood, North American Indians, who feared the specters of the first enemies they slew in battle, hoped to expiate their guilt by abstaining from sex and meat for six full months! Modern Expiators, in order to punish themselves subconsciously for supposedly "causing" the death of a loved one, may also find themselves rendered sexually impotent or frigid. This is, of course, a form of unconscious atonement not unlike the Indian superstition just described.

## Raising the Dead

The subject of ghosts and the Expiator's need to confront the dead bring us to spiritualism, a phenomenon that lucratively thrives on the superstitions now under discussion and presumes to be the one sure method of contacting the dead without further offending them or exciting their wrath. Such contact is effectuated by means of an intermediary, or medium, who usually fulfills the Conjuror-personality type discussed in the previous chapter. His, or more often her, origins go back to the necromancers of classic times, such as the witch of Endor mentioned earlier, or to the peculiar Dr. John Dee, soothsayer to Queen Elizabeth I. Such characters have surfaced in practically every country and in every age, but the officializing—or one should say systematizing—of spiritualism oddly enough came about in the 1840s in New York State. There, the teen-age Fox sisters contended that they had contacted a dead man in their farmhouse by working out a sort of Morse code with him transmitted by rappings. These ghostly sounds were later shown to have been produced by one of the sisters, who apparently could crack her toe knuckles with astonishing precision and sonority. Though the aura of fraud hung over mediumship like a fetid stench, the practice flourished, especially during the Civil War, and rappings, tappings, shrill voices, and spectral moans filled dark séance chambers from coast to coast. Led by the Fox sisters, the craze soon enveloped Europe, where the Frenchman Rivail-Kardec, a sort of psychic jack-of-all-trades, promoted his version of the anomaly called spiritism (extremely popular in South America and the Caribbean). Today, the entire movement remains a powerful quasi-religious, mystic enterprise of growing influence, less dependent these days on "things that go bump in the night" (literally) as on certain "inner" emotions and psychic "vibrations" or attitudes, manifested without the cheap theatrics of a preceding age. A typical modern séance (whether in the dark or in a lighted spiritualist church) will attempt through a medium, who may or may not be in a trance, to contact a specific control, or dead spirit, with whom previous contact has already been established. This control, by dint of his, her, or its own devices, then contacts the relative or friend being sought (it could also be Napoleon or Caesar) and relays messages back and forth like a translator at the United Nations. Rarely does the living seeker hear or see the specific "dead" person he seeks; his contact, via the medium, is only with an intermediary control—a kind of buffer to the beyond.

## The Pike-Ford Séance

The most famous and well-publicized séance in recent times (it was even televised) concerned the late Episcopal bishop of New York James Pike and a well-known psychic-spiritualist named Arthur Ford (who is currently dictating books from his niche in the afterlife). In 1967 on Canadian television Ford said he had communicated with Bishop Pike's late son through the good offices of a control named Fletcher. Ford invariably called upon this Fletcher —other mediums have used Pocahontas—who he said was a childhood chum killed in World War I. Before millions of television viewers, Fletcher-cum-Ford (or Ford-cum-Fletcher) related specific details to Pike about his son and other deceased associates, so that the bishop was thoroughly convinced that a necromantic contact had been made. At the time, rational explanations of this and similar séances could be made on the grounds of the super-suggestibility of the seeker (in this case, Pike) and the artful manner of the medium. (Ford had captured headlines in the 1920s when he asserted spirit contact with the famous magician Harry Houdini, an indefatigable debunker of mediums.)

Then in March 1973 it was widely reported that biographers of

Ford (who had died in 1971) had confessed finding in his files hundreds of obituaries clipped from newspapers that he used as references for the details he allegedly garnered from the alleged Fletcher. These obituaries included those of the very same persons Ford had discussed with Pike on television.

Very often gullible individuals are amazed or deeply impressed with the stream of facts revealed in séances which they insist no one but they—or someone dead—could possibly know. The truth of the matter is that research and trickery account for practically all such "insight" and intuition handles the rest. The Pike-Ford séance, besides its value to the necessary debunking of this sinister business —which plays on grief and fear—affords us a startling demonstration in terms of the Expiator's neurosis and susceptibility.

Bishop Pike was a deep-feeling but troubled man. Though born a Roman Catholic, he eventually rose to become a leading Episcopal prelate. Still he was often at odds with essential Christian dogma and was repeatedly accused of heresy by his peers. In 1966 he resigned his office and was censured by the House of Bishops of the Episcopal church. Thereafter, much involved with mysticism and the occult, Pike determined to retrace the paths of Christ in the Holy Land. He became lost in the Judean wilderness and died there. Among the many traumas in the bishop's life was the suicide of his son, James, Jr., in 1966 when the boy was twenty years old. The full story of this tragedy has not yet been told, but a picture emerged nonetheless of a strained relationship between father and son which might lead one to suppose a certain expiatory need on the bishop's part to unburden himself of the guilt he may have sadly assumed. Seeking out Ford, whose reputation was not exactly untarnished (the Houdini affair was left surrounded in a haze of collusion and fraud), seems to point to Pike's insecurity and inability to resolve for himself the problems entailed by his son's unfortunate death. In fact, Pike seemed bent on a type of mystic suicide himself, the ultimate irrational punishment for insupportable guilt.

## Contact with the Dead

The persistence of spiritualism and related ghostly conceits, in spite of continued and effective debunking and rational criticism, can only be laid to a deep-rooted psychological disturbance on the part of millions of people world wide, who are primarily beset by expiatory neurosis, or—to a lesser degree—by unformulated anxieties concerning death and the afterlife, which are similarly tied to feelings of inadequacy and guilt. Blatant shams, such as photographs that allege to be pictures of actual ghosts but which in most cases resemble simple inept photography or melodramatic fraud, continue to intrigue the gullible and support their superstitions. Supposedly responsible institutions and a myriad of irresponsible newspapers, magazines, and books, as well as TV personalities and supposed "experts," continue to feed the guilt anxieties of the masses regarding contact with the dead. The New York *Times*, which seems to have a predilection for the realities of occultic claims, in 1972 printed a story about "Spirit Photographs," stating that there is "a body of spirit photographs which have never been adequately explained away . . ."[4] Among these, said the *Times*, are those produced by a so-called psychic named Ted Serios, who claims to "photograph" objects solely with his eyes. Since Serios' results have been reproduced by stage magicians, there is some indication that they can indeed be "adequately explained away" in terms of trickery. Trickery also seems afoot in at least one of the alleged spirit photographs reproduced by the *Times* along with its article. It shows a veiled, transparent lady frightening two rustic gentlemen at the turn of the century and more closely resembles a scene out of a 1910-production of *Macbeth* (or some Italian opera) than anything worthy of mention in a serious publication.


## Auras and Astral Bodies

A slew of updated superstitions concerning auras, halos, astral bodies, and previous lives inflame the Expiator's imagination. Variations of these beliefs, which might be simply categorized as emanations, are universal and probably spring from Egyptian archetypes of the Ka and the animating breath of life sent forth by the creative goddess Hathor. Genesis also regards life as synonymous with breath or an airy emanation breathed by God. Kabalistic tradition, which blends the Bible with the occult, regarded vapor as essential to the "physical" form of spirits. In other words, the dead cling to the breath of life (*neshoma*) after dying in order to make themselves visible to the living on earth. Tibetan mystery cults regard this aura, or breath, as synonymous with the soul, and the mandala, the hazy circle of light and breath surrounding holy men —particularly Buddha—can be commonly seen in oriental art.

Medieval tradition idealized this optical notion in the form of a halo (or wheel) visible around the head, or, in some cases, the whole body of saints and holy persons. Christianity probably syncretized the idea from Eastern art. The figurization of the soul as an aura or halo—or astral body—led to superstitions concerning mirrors, for it was feared that these diabolic inventions (which reversed left and right) might somehow absorb the soul of one who looked into them. Breaking a mirror therefore portended a rupture of the soul and possibly death within seven years (the magic number of kabala) for those who caused the mishap.

The natural or psychological explanation of auras, halos, and mandalas may be found in the mechanics of the eye. Early sun worshipers, staring into the flaming ball which represented their god, would inevitably see "auras" or light flashes either in negative or positive form when looking back to earth, particularly at other people. The damage involved in long-term exposure of the eye to the sun, which sun worshipers would assuredly suffer, can further explain the persistence of their visions. Most theophanies, or miraculous religious conversions, take place in connection with some flaming or luminary sight: Moses and the burning bush, Paul and the blinding flash on the road to Damascus, Zoroaster's view of the clash of the demons of darkness and the god of light. Naturally, such persons who back away from their confrontations with scarred retinas or damaged sight become poor witnesses of optical truth. In addition, the average man in the ancient world was greatly amazed by reflections of himself caught in passing on a polished surface or in a pond. Such Narcissan glimpses coupled with a perennial fascination with shadows may have helped create a folklore of prototypes in which auras and ghosts are merely natural phenomena naïvely perceived.

The mystique of auras seems to imply a subsequent affirmation of the existence of ghosts, for if a man possesses an aura in life, is it not logical to assume that this entity, this presumable mass of *ectoplasm*—the fictitious substance of the soul—can then enliven itself, kabalistically perhaps, and become an astral body? Superstitiously seen, man's double or *doppelgänger*, that which goes *with* him in life, must also stand *in* for him after death. In some occultic ideas the astral body is capable of a separate identity *during* life and accounts for the visitations we presume to see in premonitions or those which are defined by kill-joy rationalists as simple hallucinations.

The aforementioned Arthur Ford experienced what he predictably viewed as an out-of-body astral projection at a time when he was in a hospital bed, critically ill. Having just been injected with a painkiller, Ford found himself "floating in the air above my bed. [I] could see my body, but had no interest in it . . . ."[5] He goes on to relate an astral visit to the Elysian Fields, in which he cheerfully visits with many old (dead) friends and even undergoes a netherworld trial as to his worthiness in the afterlife. At the critical moment, however, as the verdict is coming in, Ford is told that he must return to his body and suddenly finds himself back in his hospital bed, awakened from a two-week coma. Such a Conjuror personality as Arthur Ford, of course, could not believe himself simply a victim of natural sense alienation, resulting from a hypodermic injection. For him, the hallucination-dream becomes an astral projection and a rarified view of paradise.

Other psychics and fortunetellers have reported similar "trips," which on closer inspection resemble schizoid displacements or delusions brought about by chemical changes in the brain, either induced by medicinal drugs, by hallucinogens, or by morbid pathology. There is even another angle, according to the occultniks writing in the popular press, and this latest dimension of the astral fad is naturally concerned with sex. In fact, they call it "astral sex," in which the incorporeal emanation travels far and wide to engage in copulation with partners of a similar "vibration." To stimulate the trip, one is advised to prime the pump with a bit of masturbation in advance. In a more rational day, sex fantasies were simply —sex fantasies; not so in these Aquarian times.


## Soul Traveling and Reincarnation

Another superstition once again hotly in vogue is "soul traveling," an idea probably spurred on by a group called Eckanar, which is headquartered in Las Vegas, Nevada. Based upon Tibetan mysticism, Eckanar tries to stimulate the same out-of-body experience Arthur Ford reported in his hospital room. The process resembles kabala, in which the individual attempts to travel backward or upward from living reality, or the lower states of consciousness, to an ecstatic condition that causes him to feel unified with God. Kabalists call the levels of ascent *sephiroth;* Eckanarists refer to them as a series of "spiritual exercises," which anyone can learn for an annual fee of sixty dollars.

One man alive today has supposedly made the trip back to God successfully. His name is Darwin Gross. He lives in California, is called the living "Eck Master," and, it is reported, is leader of several million followers. According to the principles of Eckanar, Gross is part of a company that includes Jesus, Buddha, Zoroaster, Swedenborg, Napoleon, and Beethoven, among others. Also, according to press accounts, the organization's annual income exceeds 120 million dollars through sale of publications and spiritual exercises, so we can readily see the functional and financial aspects of astral superstitions. What may be more difficult to envision is how such ideas relate to the Expiator's attitude, the anxiety regarding death created by guilt, and the need to amend. Simply put, those harboring notions of revival of the dead and astral projections allow themselves, among other things, a fleeting hope that the dire finality which they believe they imposed on their loved ones will one day be lifted, that the dead will return to life in some form and then forgive their destroyers. Of course, in the interim, as ghosts or spirits, they may engage in all sorts of malicious antics. But the living demur to these in expectation of better, immortal times. For this reason, most Expiators who believe in ghosts subconsciously welcome their presence (and therefore deepen delusive beliefs) since a ghost, no matter how dreadful, promises not only an end to death, but an end to expiation and the guilt that requires it.

In tandem with such conceits is the weighty subject of reincarnation, a belief that was originally religious in form, but which is today tied closely to the fancies of the occult. In this occultic avatar, reincarnation is simply a rather subtle form of "ghostliness." But it is not the Ka, or the soul, that is of interest to those who believe in this idea. Rather they concern themselves with something called the karma, a sort of cosmic report card that memorializes the deeds of the soul as it passes through various incarnations. Compared to the ghost, who supposedly remembers his former life, the reincarnated individual does *not,* except under trance conditions or in momentary flashes along the way, because in this belief, the karma is the only connecting link between one incarnation and the next. The idea is a product of Hinduism, which regards existence as an element in a continuing cycle of retribution. Accordingly, any person walking the earth at this moment has failed to free himself from that cycle, specifically from "rebirth," because of a faulty karma. Thus the misdeeds manifested while you lived as a wealthy raja in the Vale of Kashmir are now being expiated—or should be —by your current status as a starving beggar in Calcutta. The expiatory function of the karma idea is essential to Hindu and Buddhist ethics, but it may also serve superstitious individuals as a kind of cosmic alibi for current dilemmas and injustices.

The Western interpretation of reincarnation is generally less concerned with karma, however, than it is with the conquest of death by means of rebirth and the tangential opportunity for probing the nature of death, which reincarnation supposedly affords. Those who assume they have proof of former lives, along with certain parapsychologists working in this area, seem to be almost blissfully ignorant or unconcerned with the dynamics of human psychology and neurosis when they fall upon a so-called "Bridey Murphy" case. In this phenomenon, a woman (usually), under hypnosis (always), presumes to have regressed beyond memories of her birth, back some hundred years to an obscure village somewhere in Ireland or Germany, wherever, and while entranced, reports alleged details of the former existence.

### The Case of the "Jewish" Twin

One of the most active investigators of this phenomenon is Dr. Ian Stevenson, a psychiatrist who has studied hundreds of cases which, he says, appear to point to the validity of reincarnating souls. Some of his cases swing on the flimsiest possibilities. In one, a young woman—one of identical twins—born in a typically Christian household, began to experience, around the age of eighteen, what was described as a strong attraction to Judaism. So strong was this sudden attraction that the girl insisted every Saturday upon being driven fifteen miles to a synagogue where she might pray. In talking with the subject, Stevenson learned that she believed herself in a former life to have been murdered as a Jewess by the Nazis in the 1930s. Her twin sister had no such feelings, however, so the good doctor tentatively concluded some sort of parapsychological, as opposed to psychoneurotic, explanation.

As I see it, an expiatory superstition in the form of a strong guilt neurosis was probably at play. Here a Christian girl, one of identical twins and therefore possibly seeking a new ego identity that will distinguish her from her sister, and possibly burdened by gentile guilt for the Jewish Holocaust, projects a compensatory fantasy, which she may actually believe, that she was once a Nazi victim. So strongly does she accept this idea and so willingly does she reject and degrade her present life, that she is physically revulsed by nonkosher food such as shellfish and pork.

What should be investigated in this and similar cases is not the occultic notions of reincarnation, which are more alibis than facts, but rather the possibility of neurotic guilt repression in this particular case latent anti-Semitism in the individual or in her family life. In addition, the question of possible sibling rivalry as concerns this girl should have been thoroughly explored before any fanciful leaps into karmic transmigration. The source of the subject's information about the Holocaust is also of great moment in any serious study of this case. At the very moment when this girl learned the unsettling events about Nazi brutality and concentration camps, she may have experienced some concomitant trauma, possibly sexual or pubescent in nature, which harmfully cemented the Holocaust information to her susceptible psyche. In Chapter 2, we discussed the case of a boy afflicted with what he called a "stuttering demon" and it was revealed through therapy that the sufferer had cohered the attack of a mad dog to his general insecurity and from that produced a full-blown neurotic fantasy.


## Déjà Vu


Many current examples of the reincarnation delusion (the "Expiator's Return") seem valid because of that age-old occultic sacred cow which asks: How else could so-and-so have known the obscure details he or she reported? Forgetting for the moment the fraudulent research technique, such as Arthur Ford reportedly employed, let us examine two general syndromes of this superstition in the hopes of uncovering a rational explanation for each, and at the same time, a proper perspective on the above-mentioned sacred cow.

One of the most common syndromes of the general reincarnation idea is the universal experience known as *déjà vu* (from the French for "already seen"). In this effect, the individual becomes gradually aware of a fleeting sense that "all this happened before." Such an experience may occur while he sits in a bus or at a business conference or at home watching television. The rather strained explanation of this, in occultic terms, is that we have all passed through *this* life somehow before and occasionally remember that passage. The scientific explanation concerns fatigue and altered brain chemistry, which allow the quality of memory to flow over current perceptions giving them a "second" time effect. Psychologists can simulate the *déjà vu* phenomenon in a laboratory with electrodes implanted in a volunteer's brain. There is absolutely nothing unusual or magical about this condition except to the Expiator who wishes to believe that his "guilty" life is a mysterious matter of destiny and that his actions, predetermined by some cosmic force (the karma perhaps), are not of his own responsibility.

### *"Old Souls"*

More dramatic, and far less universal than *déjà vu*, are those dramatically reported "Bridey Murphy" cases where the "old soul," or reincarnate, makes itself known under hypnosis. Early in 1975 such a case was reported in Virginia, where a minister's wife, while hypnotized, spoke in German of a former life lived in the 1870s. Superstitious people were gravely impressed with the following evidence, supplied in part by Ian Stevenson, who happens to teach at the nearby University of Virginia. The lady under hypnosis described a real village in Germany, a village she had never visited or heard about; she reported historically documented troubles in the Catholic church of the period; and above all, she spoke colloquial German, a language, she says, that she never spoke or knew in waking life. The existence of a certain town, which may be learned from any atlas, or of a historical event, available in any history book, are rather weak supports for the outlandish claims of reincarnation. Nor is the German-speaking factor at all perplexing when we learn that the subject under hypnosis is a descendant of Germans and that she may have unknowingly learned a few phrases of this fairly common language as a child. There is much evidence to show that language may be unconsciously learned (even in sleep).

What probably occurs in many cases of age regression under hypnosis is that the subject, forced back beyond birth, prefers to invent a fantasy scenario (one possibly buried in the subconscious) rather than disappoint herself or the hypnotist with a glaring blank.

Such an individual is likely to suffer from certain superstitious neuroses, particularly the Expiator's syndrome, as well as from what might be called a "Walter Mitty" imagination. By inventing another personality, usually akin to her own, the subject tries to expiate "past" guilts (which, in fact, reveal anxieties about current guilts) through the drama of a former life. Such schizoid tendencies are indicative of serious mental disorder and must be treated as such and not as some wondrous jaunt to the Hindu cosmos of birth and rebirth and the karmic wheel of destiny.

### Resurrection as Ritual

There is one more unusual consideration concerning the eventual status of the dead and that relates to resurrection. Like reincarnation, this notion is one heavily invested with religious beliefs, so much so that it is the core and turning point of the world's most influential religion, for as St. Paul says with great emphasis: "If Christ be not risen . . . your faith is vain" (I Cor. 15:17). The purpose of this book is not to investigate religious beliefs unless they are primarily superstitious ideas held for ritualistic or neurotic purposes and not for the theological and inspirational benefits they either symbolically or functionally stimulate. If belief in the resurrection of Jesus is taken as an article of faith and renewal, as an explanation of life and death and man's purpose in the universe, in short, as a religious ideal, then it stands unshakably. Jesus himself insisted to the "doubting" Thomas that those who believe without proof, thereby on faith, are far more blessed than those who require demonstration. Their faith is sufficient to the *mystical,* but not the magical, needs of religion. This pattern of transcendant and metaphysical faith is the nature of religion and the *sine qua non* of the religious mentality. With it no rational Christian goes to church to demand *or* receive a tangible demonstration of resurrection or any other miracle.

Superstitious Christians, however, do precisely that; they regard the Communion primarily as a magical act—hocus-pocus per se— and they view relics as trinkets of power and prayer as a divinational exercise. Above all, they assume that the resurrection of Christ implies the worst excesses of occultic imagination: vampires, zombies, wandering spirits, and naturally ghosts (every time they hear the expression "Holy Ghost," they shudder a little). To allay in part their superstitions, such people should know that the central event of Easter is traceable to specific pre-Christian pagan cultures and therefore should be defined as myth. The Babylonian goddess Ishtar resurrected the spring god Tammuz at the vernal equinox, and the event was celebrated throughout Europe centuries prior to Christianity; it is clearly an archetype of Easter. In fact, Ishtar is sometimes identified with Eostre, an Anglo-Saxon spring goddess, whose name is the root of the word Easter. Frazer reports that in the nineteenth century Sicilian women, among others, related Easter and the Festival of Adonis, a Syrian resurrection holiday and springtime ritual. Of this phenomenon Frazer writes: "When we reflect how often the church has skillfully contrived to plant the seeds of the new faith [Christianity] on the old stock of paganism, we may surmise that the Easter celebration of the dead and risen Christ was grafted upon a similar celebration of the dead and risen Adonis, which, as we have seen reason to believe, was celebrated in Syria at the same season."[6]

Earlier, in relation to the mythology of Satan, I tried to explain that a mark of the superstitious—that is magical—nature of a belief, may be the fact that we can trace it back to a specific cultural source—Satan to Zoroaster in Persia, for instance. In this vein, the risen Christ relates to the Syrian Adonis, who in turn derives from the Babylonian Tammuz, who himself is akin to the Phrygian worship of Attis, another deity born of a virgin and brought back to life after his death by a goddess not unlike Ishtar. Of course, the pagan sources of Christ's resurrection are often explained by Christian apologists as purposeful foreshadowings by God to prepare the way for his one true son. Investigating or debating this argument is really not within the scope of this book, except to say that when resurrectional ideas play a troublesome role in neurotic behavior, such as evinced by Expiator tendencies, and when they are employed in support of irrational conceits regarding ghosts, ghouls, and the general realm of the risen dead (or undead), then, as in previous cases, the "ghost must be laid." In this case it must be laid back to what Frazer adroitly calls a skillful contrivance on the part of the Church to win over pagan converts inculcated with resurrectional ideas, none of which Christians believe to be true in their original forms. To the person who states, therefore: If Christ was risen from the dead then why not Hamlet's father or Harry Houdini? the answer must be, it was not Christ who was risen it was Adonis, Tammuz,

Attis, Osiris, et cetera, et cetera. Will you therefore worship those ancient *pagan* gods?

But to the faithful Christian who believes in the Risen Christ as an inexplicable manifestation of God's love and power, one need not comment at all. Such a Christian, we hope, is not likely to be haunted by Hamlet's father or taken in by the claims of Arthur Ford.

## Strategies of Solace

And yet, in the face of bereavement, coping is essential, even for the most rational among us, and the strategies of solace which coping implies will include all aspects of credology, whether religious, superstitious, philosophical, or folkloric in substance. By these means we may mollify our grief and adjust to the demands that death, our own included, ineluctably portends. We must cope, however, in such terms so as to make coping bearable in itself and not a form of living death. As outlined here, the Expiator's agony and haunted mind may be often as pained and weakened in the end as the mind of him that surrenders to irreconcilable sorrow.

There is much in the realm of belief that need not necessarily ensnare us at the moment of our greatest need and which may even lead to the *summun bonum* known as peace of mind. The whole schema of winter and springtime holidays, for instance, was devised over the centuries by primitive and pagan, by Christian, Muslim, Hindu, and Jew (among others) precisely to provide such peace and solace in the face of natural and physical death. Winter's perennial gloom is brightened today by the candles of Christmas and Hanukkah, as it was in the past by the bonfires built throughout the Roman world in celebration of Sol Invictus (the Reborn or Invincible Sun). A parallel feast among Hindus is devoted to Shiva, who dances himself to a fiery death so that the world, in winter's grip, might be reborn in light. Springtime holidays, as noted in our discussion of Easter, universally recall us to life and the revival of spirit and flesh.

Superstitions as such play a relatively salutary role in these holiday reckonings with nature. May Day and April Fool's Day, for example, mark the beginning of those months in which life seems to return to the barren world—at least in the Northern Hemisphere (the usual location of the celebrations in question). Both May Day and April Fool's are rooted, superstitiously, in phallic or fertility practices. The April holiday relates to the Bacchanalias, which were wine-growing celebrations that encouraged maids and men to copulate on the barren ground in the hopes of reminding nature of its fertile powers and thus "fooling" it into activity. May Day has been identified with the Celtic festival known as Beltane, in which ithyphallic god effigies were paraded amid shows of flowers and vegetation (hence the Maypole). But crude as the origins of such holidays may seem, they bespeak a restorative, therefore commendable, fervor. The Christmas tree is no less pagan and no less magical than the Maypole, rooted as it is in the Roman Saturnalia, or winter solstice festival, and in the worship of the god Sol Invictus, who like Jesus was born on December 25 of a virgin mother. Throughout the Middle East at that date, in ancient times, fires were kindled and decorations hung ceremoniously on doorposts and trees. The eight-branched Menorah, or candelabrum, used for the Hanukkah lights in Judaism, is symbolic of the "tree of life," and this idea of a lighted tree extends to the pine forest rituals of the Teutons and Celts, to Druidism and its use of sacred mistletoe, and to the modern cheer of winter decorations. All are interrelated since all are born of the same urge, the seeking of *solace* (that is, "sol," the sun) in times of gloom.

It is good to have luminous relief during the darkness of sorrow; conversely, abnormal suppression of grief, or gloom, may eventually surface either as perennial pessimism or physical paralysis and pain. And if the grief-stricken find solace in ancient rituals or if their burdens are lightened and repressions released through funerals and wreaths, crepe hanging, and black garments—so be it. Dwelling upon sorrow even in concrete ways is functional and restoring. An amateur artist I know began painting several portraits of his recently deceased wife soon after the funeral and found that the continual confrontation with her features provided both helpful and ennobling relief. A "sort of magic," he said. In a way, his confrontation is like the common superstition that a sudden shudder down the spine indicates "someone walking over my grave" (since my grave and I shall one day be inseparable in the cold chill of silence). We are willing to relate a common physical feeling with a morbid remark because sometimes morbidity represents a type of rational defiance and a subtle unconscious attitude of realism.

## *The Courtroom of Bereavement*

Where the danger lies, as iterated throughout this chapter, is in the Expiator's crippling sense of unworthiness and guilt and in the fear these reactions promulgate. Such a person lights the memorial candles while cowering beneath phantom eyes, or dons black in the hopes of hiding from ghostly retribution, or believes himself somehow magically responsible for causing death even by a wish or an unspoken curse conceived during an emotional crisis. Psychoanalysts are continually dealing with cases of simple paralysis or dysfunction rooted in repressed beliefs concerning alleged causation of harm and death to others. Frequently an individual whose mother died giving birth to him takes upon himself an unreasonable burden of guilt and suffers a wasted life as a result. He may unconsciously attempt to expiate that "murder" by developing faulty relationships with women (or men) or by acting out his unworthiness and failure in the world and thereby actually becoming what is commonly called "a loser."

Hamlet is, of course, the ultimately haunted man, driven to expiate not his own guilt—at least not his conscious guilt—but that of his mother, with whom he so strongly identifies. Enslaved to murderous duty by the machinations of a ghost, who may yet be the devil "in a pleasing shape," the sensitive young prince slowly slips into a quagmire of gloom and death, wasting his life in deference to a phantom and to the enthrallments of his own apparent neurasthenia. No doubt, Shakespeare's play would have suffered dramatically had Hamlet merely ignored the ghost as a superstitious aberration. But how much better off poor Hamlet would have been.

Death and its anxieties are serious areas of psychology and dangerous areas where superstition is concerned, for such superstitions are often inexorably tied to irrational guilt. Therefore, it is wise when in the dim courtroom of bereavement to remember that venerable principle of Western justice that all men be deemed innocent until proven guilty. This includes each and every one of us as we judge ourselves in times of sorrow and upheaval. But as Shakespeare remarks in his greatest play: "There needs no ghost . . . come from the grave to tell us this."

CHAPTER 6

# *Cosmic Marching Orders*

The day after man's first landing on the moon, the novelist Arthur Koestler commented in the New York *Times:* "Coincident with cosmic euphoria, the world is in the grip of a cosmic anxiety."[1] Amid the apparent but quickly vanished euphoria that greeted this phenomenal lunar achievement, there was indeed, and remains, severe human anxiety, which in some cases the mysteries of outer space only help to deepen and emphasize. Ironically, for many on that epochal day in July 1969, the conquest of the moon as a triumph for science and technology was, at the same time, a defeat for the magic of the unknown and the mystical spirit of man. Like the Copernican or Darwinian revolutions, this event to them implied man's essential feebleness in the face of cosmic law. Accordingly, Neil Armstrong's "one small step" on the lunar surface was an indicator of human smallness and insecurity in the void of space—a point keenly visualized by television pictures of the planet earth receding from the Apollo lunar module like a schoolboy's marble rolling down a boulevard.

Cosmic anxiety seems to be the rule of the day; consequently, the celestial portals that were so dramatically swung open in 1969, remain, in our time, merely ajar. The majority of men, it seems, have chosen to be occupied not so much with astronomy as with astrology, not so much with the real and dynamic promise of an earthly space program as with the science fiction of UFOs. It is ironic indeed that the Space Age, with all its potential and achievement, should be one so mired in space-related superstition and error, that on the very day man landed on the moon there were those throughout the world who were doubtless far more concerned with whether the moon in conjunction with Saturn might not portend for them romantic upheaval or a melancholy mood. Today the three American astronauts who dared what was once an impossible dream are forgotten men in comparison to the so-called "gods" in their chariots, who allegedly came to earth to build landing fields on the coastal plains of South America. And the Apollo voyage itself seems dull and mechanical compared to the mystical fate of those ships and planes that dare to venture into the weird "white waters" of the Bermuda Triangle.

Pablo Picasso commenting, like Koestler, in the New York *Times* on July 21, 1969, spoke for many about the lunar landing when he said, "It means nothing to me. I have no opinion about it and I don't care."[2] At least the famous painter was unequivocal. Those persons whom I call Stargazers, who relate earth-bound anxieties to the alleged magic of outer space, ostensibly agree with Picasso, but in their hearts they are really saying: "I didn't want this to happen. It may eventually disprove the mysterious influence of the moon on the flow of my blood and therefore upon my emotions. It may reduce the goddess Diana to a lump of sterile clay. True, the Aquarian Age implies wonder and adventure and far-reaching exploration, but not the type of exploration that will destroy our myths and dreams. Don't tell me astrology is unscientific and out of step with astronomy. Don't disprove for me the hope that beings from another world will one day descend on our pitiful planet and save us from our anxieties. Aquarius is a giver of dreams, a sustainer of illusions, not someone who strips away the veil of mystery and leaves us naked in the ice-cold climate of space."

Speaking on television in Syracuse, New York, in 1975, a lady UFO expert said she looked forward to a landing some time soon of "350 million space ships from some ninety other universes," which will come here to help us out of our "mass karma thing," that is, our problems concerning war and poverty and drugs and the high price of gasoline. "I'd feel lost," said the "expert," without "my hope in the UFOs."[3]

"We are adrift in a sea of space," an astrologer once told me. "Our only dependable guidelines are the stars." A cleaning lady I formerly employed was of the same opinion in a less poetic manner. She would sometimes call early in the morning of the day she was supposed to come to my house to report that "it wouldn't work," meaning her horoscope for that day wouldn't work and therefore neither would she. "If I do come in, something valuable is going to break," she once told me.

"For those of my readers who are unaware of these things and think that I am exaggerating," wrote Carl Gustav Jung some twenty years ago, "I can point to the easily verifiable fact that the heyday of astrology [and all cosmic superstitions] was not in the benighted Middle Ages, but is in the middle of the twentieth century . . ."[4]

Much has been written—by Jung and others—about the astrology explosion in modern times and the millions of dollars spent world wide on horoscopes, charts, Zodiac emblems, and other such accouterments, and we are all aware of the latest trends concerning UFOs, space visitors, vibrations from cosmic forces, and so on. We are equally cognizant, or should be, of the debunking that of necessity always accompanies astrologic and magically cosmic claims. But what we have in the main failed to grasp are the psychological roots of insecurity that feed stargazing, or cosmic, superstitions. Recognizing such roots need not demean or reprove those who cling to them, nor is ridicule our aim. But assessing, on the one hand, the very human and explainable insecurities that lead to cosmic fallacies and, on the other hand, understanding the anti-scientific origins of these allegedly scientific ideas may go a long way to reducing the dependency, and therefore the danger, that any one of us faces when we rely on delusion. The *ignis fatuus* (the fool's fire) that beckoned ancient man in the forests primeval and often turned out to be ignited swamp gas or fireflies may still command a certain fascination (as does the Zodiac and the ubiquitous UFO), but fascination need not lead to enslavement. After all, those who darted in pursuit of the *ignis fatuus* often found themselves fallen in a bog with nothing to reach for but the distant stars.


### As Above, So Below


The current interest in cosmic magic may be divided into two apparently opposite areas. First, the astrological, which deals with visible cosmic elements, and secondly, space, per se, which deals with the invisible and essentially unknown. Both have developed superstitiously out of the tandem beliefs that the macrocosm, or the sky, mirrors by magical design the microcosm, or man's world, on the ancient theory, "As it is above so below." The single most resonant chord that such a philosophy strikes is the inherent insecurity that everyone feels when "adrift" in both his own microcosm and in the teleological macrocosm. The eternal question in this regard has always been how to handle this very human insecurity; in short, how to cope? Those who turn to the heavens for the answers believe these answers lie buried (but not hidden) in the macrocosm and that when properly uncovered will afford the drifter a set of unbeatable marching orders that promise tranquillity, success, and the same sort of security he might feel in his mother's arms.

Besides the teleological dimension, there is another ironic aspect of cosmic delusions that presumably affords security and hope. I speak of the quasi-scientific nature that surrounds astrology and UFOs and invests them with apparently respectable, easily provable, and ultimately *anti*magical qualities. When astrologers talk of conjunctions, sextiles, orbits, degrees, and so forth, they are utilizing the very same jargon as their unfriendly counterparts, the astronomers. Similarly, most books and lectures concerned with the more egregious aspects of UFOs and the like are steeped in aerodynamics, physics, mathematics, and space-lab technology. The Stargazers of either category view themselves, in fact, as the "scientists" of the "unknown." They deplore most associations with the occult and often sneer at witchcraft, Ouija boards, and shrug their shoulders regarding questions of demon possession and visitations from the dead. Indeed, there is some truth to the assertion that Stargazers, by comparison, are the more rationalistic of all other superstitious types because they relate to systems, rules, and what appear to be rational conclusions. This relationship, ironically, is endemic to personal insecurity, which, as a psychological problem, often drives the individual to the most rigid sorts of formulas and procedures that frequently have the veneer of significance. Carried to its extreme, such insecurity may lead to a paranoic condition. Psychotherapists report that the typical paranoid demonstrates highly perceptive, systematized attitudes toward the stimuli of his disorder. His imagined enemies are clearly labeled and described; his methods for handling them equally formalized. In fact, he goes about his business with an enviable aplomb, amid fussy details and labyrinthian designs.

For his part, the average person, excessively insecure about an intended car trip, provides himself with a stack of road maps, directions, and instructions. People caught in the commonplace throes of job or marital insecurity likewise devise "programs" and procedures in terms of appearance, speech, and interpersonal activity so that they may overcome their fears. Often these are helpful—so long as they are rooted in reality. An up-to-date road map of an unfamiliar area will very likely provide a traveler—insecure or otherwise—with valuable assistance. But if the road map is wrong, out of date, or inaccurate, he may end up going south where he should go north and like those who pursue the *ignis fatuus* land up eventually in a bog.

### *Astronomy and the Sun Signs*

Astrology falls into the superstitious-occultic category precisely because it is essentially a faulty road map of the sky. A system it is, to be sure, and a seemingly scientific system with hundreds of rules and regulations. But when examined in terms of its essential *astronomical* premises, it shows itself to be as delusory as spiritualism, as enthralled as witchcraft, and as semantically naïve as the business of amulets and talismans. If it therefore functions and works as far as its followers believe, then it must do so by means of magic, for it does not do so by science and fact. On March 21, the vernal equinox of this year and for the last two thousand years or so, the sun aligned (or "rose") with the earth in the Zodiac field of Pisces, not Aries as most astrologers insist. This means that progressively (or precessionally) each sun sign, or nativity period, is off in the popular horoscopes by about thirty days. Astronomically this is an undeniable fact, although astrologers can finesse it quite cleverly, as we shall see. As such, this fact throws a cosmic-sized monkey wrench into all astrological calculations, for if the stars and planets affect human conditions as all Stargazers by definition believe, then the wrong stars in the wrong place reduce these calculations to inevitable error even as the faulty road map turns north into south. An astrologer tells his client, born on July 4, 1940, for instance, that the sun "rose" that day in Cancer, with Venus "rising" in Scorpio. This therefore means such and so. The such-and-so part not withstanding, astronomers scientifically can prove that on July 4th, 1940, the sun stood in relationship to Gemini (the sun, as every good Copernican knows, does not rise) and Venus stood in relationship (Venus also doesn't rise—*or* fall) to Libra. What this may mean in terms of human fate and personality is irrelevant if the relationships to begin with are wrong.

It is perfectly possible that celestial bodies have some sort of electromagnetic effect (not influence, but *effect*) on earth and its inhabitants. That these are specific and primary psychological effects, such as amatory, intellectual, or emotional, is very dubious. But even if they are, imagine how many billion celestial bodies exist (far more than the Zodiac and the planets) and what kind of Gargantuan system would be required to analyze and apply each of these factors; it boggles the mind. Furthermore, even if they do affect us, all these billion bodies, how can they do so if incorrectly calculated?

Astrologers hasten to report that they are aware of the precessional shift that has pushed the stars thirty degrees westward (or downward) in the Zodiac, causing Cancer to move into the area formerly occupied by Leo; Gemini to evict Cancer, Taurus evict Gemini, et cetera. But, say these "modern" practitioners, astrology deals with the signs (or houses), not with the actual stars, and whereas the *stars* of Gemini may now be in the area where Cancer's stars once resided, the *sign*—or name—Cancer, for some magical reason, still applies and with it all its alleged influences. This is like saying that one can still see baseball games at the site of Ebbet Field in Brooklyn, even though the stadium has long since been demolished.

## *Historical Astrology*

The delusory nature of astrology, and therefore its superstitious dimension, is further revealed by its historical development from the celestial temples of ancient Babylon to the horoscope columns of the daily press. Stargazing per se was a religious practice among the Babylonians, who developed a class of celestial magicians, the Chaldeans, in order to chart their heavens and the apparent movement of their gods. Babylonian astrology differed from the modern practice in explicit use, for the Chaldeans were not concerned with predictive, or horary, influence as much as with the seasonal appearance of their gods (the planets) and the relationships of these erratic beings to the agricultural prosperity of the nation. Observation of celestial movements as well as navigational charting became the earnest science of astronomy in ancient Greece. Greek precursors of modern astronomy, like Hipparchus, for instance, were unconcerned with the alleged occultic influences of the stars and planets and directed their efforts to interpreting correctly the movements of heaven and earth. Hipparchus, in fact, discovered precession (and thus obliterated astrology) as early as 130 B.C., but his revamping of the Zodiac in accordance with the calendar was not integrated with the astrological scheme of the day, a scheme based on Chaldean empiricism.

It was in Rome around 300 B.C. that this system of astrology was "officialized" (along with the Roman names we use today). At that point in time, the sun was in fact aligned with Aries at the vernal equinox (March 21). As fate would have it, a precessional shift occurred sometime between 300 B.C. and Hipparchus' observations in 130 B.C., correctly placing Pisces at March 21. To the Romans, who first packaged modern astrology, the signs and the stars were identical and they would have probably altered their charts had they been aware of Hipparchus' work. But they were not. And in the second century A.D., when Ptolemy of Alexandria fixed the rules of astronomy and astrology in his *Almagest*, precession was discounted as was the heliocentric nature of the solar system—also hinted at by Hipparchus.

For thousands of years, during all this astrological scheming, earth had remained the center of the universe. There was enough insecurity in the world without detaching man and his base from its supersignificant place. In this place even the great god Sol (the sun) rose and set in obedience to Mother Earth. This was also true of the fickle (ergo emotional) moon and all other visible wanderers (the Greek word for which is *planetes*).

As noted, the Chaldeans had identified these erratic movers with their gods. The Greeks followed suit and the Romans simply latinized the Hellenic names. These mythic names, which we use today, in themselves are quintessential in the superstition of astrology. In fact, without them, the particular influence ascribed to each body in relation to mankind would not exist. Stargazers, of course, believe that the name was somehow magically applied, fixing the influence as a godly prerogative. Less starry-eyed individuals may find the following causation more convincing. Because the little wanderer closest to the sun moved rapidly like a courier, clearly he should be called Mercury, courier of the gods, and as such, his mercurial activity should influence (by poetic logic) mercurial activities among men, such as wit, travel, finances, and health (which may go up or down). That planet which appears earliest in the evening, "out on the street" so to say, and returns home in the dawn, "the last one in," clearly must be the love (or lust) goddess Venus, influencer of love, sensation, and beauty. Dripping blood—at least his ruddy hue looks like a bloody glow—Mars, the war god, stimulates—because of his proverbial attributes—courage and belligerence and similar bellicose inclinations.

This poetic wordplay technique applies as well to the constellations of the Zodiac, that ecliptical belt of stars through which—so it appears to us on earth—the planets move. Like the wanderers, these star clusters are similarly creatures of mythology, and like the planets, their names also stimulate their alleged attributes. Unfortunately, modern astrologers, by and large, are unaware of the classic, therefore "authentic," origins of the Zodiacal names, thus ascribing erroneous meanings to the likes of Pisces, Cancer, Taurus, Sagittarius, and so forth. One very popular modern astrologer, for instance, wrote: "You won't find Cancer pursuing fame with passion —he pursues nothing with true passion . . ."[5] Yet the crab called Cancer by the Romans was the passionate and fearless creature who assisted Hercules in his fight with the Hydra and who, for his valor, was placed among the stars by Juno, queen of the gods. The true astrological effect of Cancer (whose actual dates are, according to astronomy, July 21–August 15) should be that of fearless bravery, hot pursuit, and courage (perfect for Napoleon, who was actually born when the sun was in the "claw end" of Cancer on August 15). Similarly, Capricorn is not merely a goat, but rather the feisty earth-god Pan in disguise (January 22–February 22), nor is Taurus simply a bull, but rather Zeus, or Jupiter, transformed into a bull for the purpose of an amorous adventure.

Without the proper knowledge of accurate celestial positions and the traditional meanings of astral names, astrology is as pointless as tightrope walking without a rope. Even a "corrected" system (as I mischievously advanced in an enterprise called *Sky Diamonds: The New Astrology*) does not change the premise. Astrology basically remains a superstition, since it would depend in any form on myths and magic formulas long since depropagandized. We at long last know, for example, that the body called Mars does not drip blood and therefore might as well be called Gandhi or XYZ and give off "peaceful" emanations. In fact, the Chinese have a whole set of different names for the same stars and planets and, accordingly, an entirely different system for calculating events and ascribing effects.

## Moonglow and Lunacy

Even the moon, the very body on which men have stood since 1969, is endowed with alleged cosmic properties that derive from purely superstitious notions long ago disproved. And yet how many Stargazers and others today regard the moon with almost unquestioning attitudes as to its influence on crime, lunacy, love, the flow of blood, the transformation into monsters, and its source as a way station for galactic visitors. No doubt there is some security provided for the more timid Romeos and Juliets among us by knowing that the "inconstant moon" is safely ensconced in the sky available for amorous or poetic stimulations. To prove this power, romantics especially point to the alleged increase of sexual activity and "necking" in lover's lanes on the night of a full moon. How precisely such statistics are obtained without one falling victim to accusations of voyeurism, I'm not sure. Suffice it to say that the full moon obscured by clouds and rain would simply have no such effect, because it is the *sight* of the glowing, silvery orb and not its inherent radiational powers that causes romantic notions, particularly in lover's lanes.

The compendium of superstitions about the moon's reputed powers existing in the modern imagination is largely based on a misinterpretation of the moon's magnetic causation of tides, which asserts that because the moon (forming a magnetic field with the sun) has a gravitational pull on the earth, it follows that this same pull should be significant where humans are concerned. Some superstitious persons even believe that female menstrual cycles are governed *uniformly* by the twenty-eight-day phases of the moon, and that the full moon is therefore a troublesome time for universal womanhood. While it is true that magnetic forces are manifested by the moon (and other celestial bodies), it is also true that electromagnetic radiation literally bombards the earth (men and women included) from myriad sources, including gas clouds, nuclear explosions, radio beams, sunlight, lasers and masers, and other human bodies. The doctor who delivers a baby has a stronger magnetic effect on the infant than the heavenly stars. The nearest one (besides the sun) is called Alpha Centauri, and it is about 25 *trillion* miles away!

Naturally, the periodicity of the moon has afforded a comforting celestial calendar since ancient times, announcing time, festivals, and seasonal shifts. In this friendly and dependable way, it is indeed a wonderful entity and, when full, a welcome field of light in the countryside. But insecurity can pervert even the best aspects of nature. In the Middle Ages, those who could not medically explain insanity, epilepsy, and such outrages as child abuse and murder tended to look toward the same luminous, seasonal (or tidal) changes in the universe as stimuli for earthly disorder. Because of the moon's compelling appearance and frequent alteration, superstitious man easily related the disappearance of the moon to the birth of demons and monsters, and by poetic logic a full moon implied tumescence, turgidity, and other concepts of bursting—murder among them. The crescent moon was seen as a sword, or as a sign of fertility and burgeoning power. (For this reason it was adopted by Islam as a symbol of militant realization.) The new moon, which is naturally not visible, signified evil, secrecy, the Sabbat of witches and sorcery. Naïve people believe the moon actually changes in shape during its phases, an idea which intensifies their faith in its magical powers. We know today that the amount of sunlight reflected from the moon creates the *illusion* of waxing and waning. The actual body itself undergoes no alteration, as any astronaut who's been there can tell you.

Even so, those today, as in the past, who tend to transfer personal responsibility outside themselves, find in the moon a perfect alibi for neurotic emotions and sudden moods or antisocial activities. "I can't be with people tonight," such an individual rationalizes; "the moon is full and I'm all jumpy and tense." The same person will probably feel secretive and bewitching in the dark of the moon by virtue of similar poetic casuistry. To test the alleged influences of the full moon, or any moon, on crime (another superstitious alibi which most people believe), I obtained statistics in Manhattan and Brooklyn for violent crimes during the period of one year for the months January, April, August, and November. There was absolutely no discernible pattern in relation to the phases of the moon. The only operative factor that affected street violence was heavy rainfall, which sometimes "wiped it out" (when the rain forced people to stay indoors) and sometimes encouraged it (as muggers preyed on isolated persons blindly hurrying home through wet, deserted streets). In August and November, at the full-moon period, an element of superstition did apparently tend to cause disturbances, not because of any physical powers of the moon, but rather, owing to psychological clichés: a large, bright moon equals "trouble." In January of the year I studied, the full moon was obscured by clouds and no variance was notable, even with so called "lunatics."

And so, whether made of green cheese (as Erasmus quipped) or sterile clay (as the astronauts assert), the moon for all its electromagnetic output remains magical more in the eye of the beholder than in actual testable fact and owes more to poetry and self-fulfilling prophecy than to science for its "moony" effects.

### Wordplay in Horoscopes

Naïve semantics, which cause the moon to be "moony," are indispensable to astrology, as noted, and therefore function well in the Stargazer's need for ordered perceptions and unswerving truths. He will find these disciplines even in the most evasive and vaguely worded horoscopes, so long as some aspect of the general sun sign and planetary ideal is upheld—no matter how feebly or how poorly researched. Thus Scorpio is always invested with a certain sexual implication, which even the celibate or prudish Scorpion may integrate into his beliefs, particularly when the terminology is cleverly finessed. *Cosmopolitan* magazine, which, like most female-directed publications, runs an astrological column, predictably reports that Scorpio's passions "run from the spiritual to the morbidly decadent."[6]

I once conducted a test in a class of fifty people. Utilizing an IBM print-out horoscope, I obliterated the pertinent word (Cancer), made twelve Xerox copies, and then typed in on each of the twelve a different sun sign name (Aris, Pisces, etc.). I then asked ten volunteers who were Pisces, Aries, Taurus, and so forth to read what he thought to be his natal horoscope and then answer the following questions by percentile: Do you think this horoscope fits your personality (80–100 per cent, 50–80 per cent, 20–50 per cent, etc.)? Do you feel this horoscope fits the way other people see you (same percentages)? In each and every case the questions were answered in the 80–100 per cent bracket, and no wonder. The opening sentence of the print-out began: "You are a creature of contrasts with a pronounced double nature . . ." The double nature concerned a tack toward capricious fantasy, on the one hand, and a need for creature comforts, on the other. Since this sort of sophistry applies to practically every one of us, I wasn't surprised with the unanimous ratings. The students, I should add, were, in fact, greatly surprised when they learned they had been "swindled" by my test. So-called "scientific," as opposed to popular, astrology is no less evasive and far more pedantic. A paper called *The Aquarian Agent* reporting on the findings of the "Association for Research in Cosmecology" discussed "an astrological study of coronary heart disease" and concluded, among other things, that "certain planets making certain aspects to other planets were found to be anywhere from very significant to highly significant . . . Mars square the sun was one of these, but we adjusted the orbs to 9 degrees forming and 6 degrees separating in order to emphasize the difference most strikingly."[7] How comforting for the hypochondriac—*if* he can figure it out.

Astrology has always devised evasive ways of handling the so-called definitive attributes of each sign and planet. This is especially true concerning physical appearances and health prognoses like the one above, all of which are fairly mutable depending on one's rising or falling factors, the ascendant sign—which connotes facial type—cusps, negative traits, positive traits, neutral traits, and so forth.

## *Astrology and Mental Health*

But as said earlier, debunking astrology is not the essential purpose of this chapter. We are concerned with the psychological origins of this superstition and its beneficial or harmful effects. In this context, astrology fulfills the following systematic functions in the Stargazer's syndrome—all related in some way to self-confidence, identity, and a sense of security in the flux of time and space.

1.) *Astrology as an ego trip.* In this aspect, the believer hopes to learn what specific personality characteristics may be expected of him according to date and place of birth. This information is then applicable, willy-nilly, to all facets of his life: career, romance, family, health, and social responsibility. Further, because astrology so greatly emphasizes celebrity status, the individual not only discovers his own dynamics and weaknesses but is impressed with the fact that a well-known movie star or athletic figure shares these identical traits, thus bolstering his faith in them. Ego building may beneficially result from these rules and regulations of identity so long as such rules are merely jumping-off points for self-analysis and development. Unfortunately, the delimiting problems of such identity dependence should be self-evident. Erich Fromm, discussing what he calls pseudo-thinking (which astrology may be), warns that the problem in it is "whether the thought [produced] is the result of one's own thinking . . ."[8] as opposed to the concoctions of an astrologer who never met the individual. Ego tripping in astrology, as a result, precludes "one's own thinking" and leads to compulsive tendencies. "I am an aggressive Capricorn, like Richard Nixon; therefore I must or should [consciously or unconsciously] act accordingly." By extension, those dominated—and captivated—by the aggressive notions of Capricorn or the vacillations of Gemini may just as easily believe themselves "shrewd" if they are Jewish, "stingy" if Scottish, "rhythmic" if black, or any other such vapid canard.

Astrology addicts must ask themselves if they are willing to risk unconscious capitulation to such facile pseudo-thinking in exchange for the dubious comforts of stereotypic identity. And if this general question is unconvincing, let them also ask whether, in addition to the various celestial positions, they are willing to reckon the not-so-ego-vaunting importance of genetic and hereditary factors in their parents, or the influence of infant environment, of schooling, health and early toilet training. Will a baby with rickets who was born of an unwed mother, if he happens to be a Sagittarian, invariably be athletically or physically motivated (as Sagittarians sre supposed to be)? And if not, why seek out rules and regulations that are consistently variable, when in fact, free development is the essence of a healthy ego identity?

2.) *Astrology as a crystal ball*. Predictive astrology presumes to provide specific answers via its systematized calculations concerning a wide range of prognoses, among them health, success, and interpersonal expectations. These prophecies may be homiletic and vague—such as those in the daily papers—or, when charted to the individual in an elaborate, "personalized" scheme, tend to take on the quality of specificity and detail. One popular astrologer flatly stated that persons born on certain dates in 1951 will all have suffered a broken finger by the age of five! (The one person in ten thousand who did is awed by the prophecy and dutifully reports the miracle far and wide, giving credence to the superstition.)

Whether specific or generalized, predictive astrology may be a very comforting ploy for those suffering the usual forms of insecurity neurosis. Hypochondria, a classic form of insecurity, is particularly indulged because astrology, since the Middle Ages, has attempted to relate sun signs and planets to various parts of the body in terms of health. Thus, those born in Cancer, who are probably already traumatized by the dreaded name of their sign, are told to expect difficulties in the lungs and chest (sometimes the stomach), which are for some reason "governed" by the Crab. If the astrological warnings about illness in these areas tend to make the Cancerian more cautious about drafts and smoking, all well and good. The trouble is that in predictive matters, astrology, like all other related superstitions, very often *creates* rather than predicts the eventualities and sets up a fatalistic mechanism that impedes free action and will. This is especially true when we realize that Stargazers tend to be insecure to begin with and therefore prey to psychological and psychosomatic ills. Accordingly, when the superstitious Cancerian learns that lung trouble or stomach cancer is his probable fate according to the stars and charts and ancient formulas, his first reaction will not be preventative and self-protective; he will more than likely experience an uncanny sense of submission. An irony of the insecure syndrome is its need to be subtlety sustained; therefore nullification of anxieties often deprives the neurotic individual of the ironic security his insecurities themselves provide! He may therefore think: "As surely as I am sensitive and domesticated because of my Cancer origins, so it must follow that I will soon develop difficulties in breathing or symptoms of asthma. I'd rather this wouldn't be, but at the same time, if it fails to occur, it may mean that my entire horoscope is faulty. I do not wish to sacrifice the over-all guarantees of astrology or the many positive things my chart predicts; therefore I must submit to the 'divine' decision and hope for the best." Considering the emotional basis of most asthmatic conditions, it can be seen how such unconscious "reasoning" can lead to the process of self-fulfilling prophecy and psychosomatic asthmatic attacks.

The same self-fulfilling can be true as regards other aspects of predictive astrology; the tall, dark stranger, the conflicts on the job, the clashes in marriage—most of these can be materialized by unconscious maneuvers in aid of "securing" the insecure.

3.) *Astrology as a substitute religion.* As noted, astrology began as a religious ideal in Mesopotamia. Its divinatory influence can be seen in the Bible and in medieval Christian adaptiveness, which embraced the Zodiac, transforming the twelve pagan sun signs into the twelve apostles. Even so, traditional religion has not encouraged this belief and, conversely, believers in it have not been encouraged by traditional religion. In fact, for them, the rules and regulations of astrology more than suffice as a religious ideal and are preferable to the usual churchy rituals and dogma. Ritualistically, astrology may indeed offer more in specific detail than any current religion. Besides, the regimen is entirely analogous to a religious code. Morning prayers, for instance, in this substitute faith are enacted by a quick look at the daily horoscope published in the local gazette or a quick call to one's personal astrologer. Carroll Righter, the *doyen* of Hollywood astrologues, reports that several of his superstar clients do not even get out of bed before dialing his hotline for a quotidian homily. In this same way, astrology may also be a form of substitute psychotherapy, which in some cases is also in itself a form of substitute religion.

Once morning prayers are intoned, the Astrologian (as opposed to Christian) places around his neck the religious symbol of his faith, the appropriate Zodiac symbol, deferring as ever to his god or gods (in this case, the Roman pantheon of planets). He then may proceed to his "confessor" (astrologer) for a personalized charting session, all the while enacting the tenets of his belief—avoiding a Scorpio if he is an Aquarian just the way an Orthodox Jew avoids pork. Or he may purchase so many shares of XYZ, Inc. because the corporation promises spectacular earnings as a result of being "born" under a favorable conjunction of Jupiter and Leo.

Astrologians celebrate religious holidays, or periods, which inspire their faith, such as the seven-year Uranian cycles and the Aquarian Age. They congregate for worship at seminars and schools, venerate sages and "priests," some of whom have become quasi-religious demigods, like the American Evangeline Adams or

Madame Soleil in France, and in a manner identical to most fundamentalist piety, they insist upon the absolute truth of their revelation and attempt to proselytize the unenlightened.

William James did not include astrology among his varieties of religious experience, but he might as well have, since it does—all jesting aside—fulfill his definitions of pragmatic and spiritual needs, with one essential difference. A skeptic may debunk Judaism, Catholicism, or Christian Science in terms of plausible and probable discrepancies concerning faith ("Moses did not part the Red Sea, it's a myth"), to which the religious person will say: "Belief in God implies that God can and might do anything." In short, faith defends against skepticism and criticism. In astrology, the attack is not so much against the faith of the believer as it is against his *facts*. Venus does not rise or descend in actuality, only in visual relation to the revolutions of the earth. The constellation Taurus is an arbitrary designation consisting of thousands of stars light-years apart from each other with no testable or provable emanating influence on human personality. The variations in time of birth for persons in the Northern Hemisphere are meaningless, considering the vastness of space et cetera. In other words, the Astrologian religion can be challenged not only by skeptics, but by experts in the business of celestial information, to wit, astronomers, 99 per cent of whom challenge it.

The psychological problem of what I earlier called "the paper crutch" therefore ensues. Those who have adopted astrology as a substitute religion unconsciously or instinctively know that it is open to a barrage of logical attacks endangering their dependence on it and more so demeaning them in the eyes of family and friends. It is unwise to lean on a paper crutch, especially if your ankles are already swollen. It is far more risky to place one's emotional faith in a system so frequently and easily challenged.

But then again, the Stargazer syndrome as outlined here inherently craves a certain amount of risk and secretly attempts to ensure the anxieties of insecurity, since these anxieties are at least dependable as recognizable, habitual, albeit uncomfortable, verities in an otherwise drifting existence.

4.) *Astrology as a Cop Out.* Most Stargazers do not become pious Astrologians, that is, religiously fanatical believers, and this may be not so much because they harbor inner doubts about their faith as it is for the more psychological reason that they cling to astrology merely as a buffer between them and the real world. They only believe in astrology as it suits their immediate emotional needs, mostly in a negative way. In modern jargon this propensity is called the "cop out," a sort of internalized game in which the player may point to the heavens as a scapegoat for his own inabilities or mistakes. Two sorts of people rely on astrology for cop-out reasons: those with a great deal of responsibility and an equal amount of insecurity, and those deemed to be losers, who avoid responsibility because of the insecurities with which they've been raised. The first type often employs astrology in a creative way, constructing celestial alibis to prevent latent insecurity from overwhelming the job, i.e., "I will not walk off the set today even though I'm uncertain about this film. I'm a Capricorn with Mars rising and I work best under pressure and jibes." Of course, even this creative utilization of astrology can degenerate into a cop out, since the individual, having now relegated his abilities to external causes, concurrently faces the problem that the slightest changes in those causes can reverse his fate, i.e., "Today Mars is in conjunction with Saturn; I'll probably have an awful day. Better call the studio and tell them I'm sick."

Admittedly, this sort of reversal doesn't happen as frequently with successful believers, who tend to master their insecurities as part of their success. Astrology, like the lion's share of superstitions, appeals most often to those who cannot master their fates and therefore seek an alibi to excuse their maladjustment. ("I'm a Capricorn with Mars rising. That's why I'm always being unfairly pressured and ridiculed . . .") One of the perennial cop-out devices of astrological belief is the negative-positive interpretations one may give to the generalizations in horoscopes or charts. To the "winner," a Pisces ascendant means a "strong demeanor, rich in expression"; to a loser, "the face of a fish." Indeed physical or inherent characteristics, which those plagued by insecurity take to be the attributes of a crushing fate, are often facilely explained by astrology, for it not only governs health but also soma-type, race, sexual preference, and appetite. Accordingly, the strong appeal of astrology to offbeat groups and minorities, to the disenchanted young, and to people groping their way is proverbial—and played to by astrologists and horoscope columns.

The agonizing problem with the cop-out ploy in this or any other superstition is that it does not usually improve the lot of those who employ it, and, in fact, may deepen insecurity and the loser's formation of neuroses. Career and marriage are most susceptible in this area. A person finds himself, for instance, unable to work with someone because he's a negative Sagittarian ("bossy, crude"), or he enacts a prophesied marital crisis apparently reported in the horoscope columns or implied in charts or other "documentary" and supposedly personalized literature. Naturally, astrologers are the first to warn us that "the stars impel; they do not compel." But the susceptibility factors in those who tend to cop out or withdraw or suffer self-defeat and anxiety are far too well developed to be merely impelled by anything. Compulsion, in fact, is a standard by-product of anxiety, ambivalence, and insecurity, and according to psychotherapists, is often involuntary under stress, a sort of knee-jerk reaction that invades the deepest functions of the body and mind. For those who compulsively seek to avoid responsibilities, to wallow in self-defeat, to blame God, nature, and man for their fate, astrology offers a perfect gambit. It is, for such persons, a *deus ex machina*, who descends on the drama of their lives to resolve, usually in a negative way, what they can not. Sadly, this god has long since lost his divinity and the mechanism that lowers him on stage is feeble and likely to snap.


## *Game Playing*

There are other common psychological functions of astrology that overlap with the ones just discussed. One significant aspect falls into the category of "Games People Play," as outlined by the late Dr. Eric Berne. In the Stargazer's game one plays generally alone, with himself and his celestial reckoning. Typical of this maneuver is the trick of allowing the chart or horoscope to "decide" what you really want it to decide—buying an expensive bauble, taking a particular trip, or calling someone out of the past. It's a fairly harmless game except that it deepens externalization of personality, at least in the conscious level. Another bit of astrological game playing relates to the ego-trip factor and might be called, in the manner of Berne, "My sign is better than yours." It is probably a conceit of all twelve Zodiac shibboleths, although Scorpios and Aquarians are usually the most envied for their alleged high planes of excitement. In tandem with this deference to arrogance is the game of "I don't believe in it, but it seems to work." In this, the assumedly logical and unsuperstitious individual is nevertheless amazed by the "accuracy" of his horoscope in terms of personality traits, quirks, habits, and the like, which a given horoscope reports about his birthday period. By and large such people are easily satisfied or carelessly gulled by references to "sensitivity, secret passions, high moral ideas, a craving for sweets (or luxuries)," and similar universal inclinations. How would these impressionable folks react to a horoscope that contained specifics such as "secret racial bigotry and voyeuristic masturbatory preferences"? Even if true, most people would resent such slurs and dutifully ignore them.

The roulette game variation of astrology should not be overlooked in this summary. It touches on risk factors common to attitudes of insecurity and shows itself at times of critical choice: "Shall I move; quit my job, buy this lottery ticket?" Where a gamble is implied, those inclined may check with the stars to help them decide. If they really want to move or quit, of course, the horoscope will invariably allow it. If not, they will bow to the warning of the sky. Either decision could be inferred from the following celestial advice taken from a prominent New York newspaper: "A chance for change should be looked upon as meaningful and decisive this year." Meaningful and decisive—but how?

And finally, there is the ever-lurking tendency among those who view the world as a threat simply to adopt current styles and fads as a lifebuoy maneuver. One might call this the "Bandwagon" effect: "Get aboard, everybody is." And considering the millions of astrology advocates and reminders that exist these days throughout the world, from the Zodiac sweepstakes held annually in France to the astrologically sanctioned coronation in 1975 of King Birendra in Nepal, how can any sensible person eschew the trend, especially if he is an Aries with Leo in ascendance, Mars in conjunction with Mercury, Jupiter square Venus, Mars trine Saturn, and the sun undergoing a total eclipse?

## Identifying the Unidentified

We should now turn back to the sky as an ineffable void of mystery and not as a map of specific destiny and type. In this context, we will be dealing with superstitious attitudes concerning what are generally known as Unidentified Flying Objects (although Stargazers identify them readily as interplanetary visitors) and such Sci-Fi related notions as gods from outer space, the lost kingdom of Atlantis (an innerspace idea, so to speak), the Bermuda (and other) Triangle, and the general mythology of the spooky sky. I am concerned with these concepts in terms of the psychology of superstition because they often foster magical, that is occultic, explanations that tend to be taken in the same irrational vein as the subjects previously rehearsed. By no means does this imply that all opinions concerning UFOs are to be lumped as superstitions. Sober and unemotional views of extraordinary "spacecraft" in our skies, including those conducted by government agencies; geologic explanations for what might have been Atlantis; and certain aspects of both the Chariot of the Gods and Bermuda Triangle stories are ostensibly tolerable as rational conjecture and investigation. But enthralling descriptions of mythic spacemen, the underwater control of destiny manifested by the buried continent of Atlantis, and supernatural interpretations of the giant pyramid vis-à-vis ancient gods simply cater to the insecurities we have been discussing. They do so by rather seductively appealing to those who feel adrift in a celestial data bank and who therefore need assurances that extraterrestrial forces will very shortly put all things right.

## *Little Green Men*

A certain fancy for fairy tales and fairy godmothers permeates these conceits and often goes hand in glove with a lack of earthbound interests and a strong dose of fundamentalistic cant. The UFO expert from Syracuse, New York, earlier mentioned, who appeared on television to announce the imminent landing of 350 million spacecraft (invisible) that will thwart an atomic Armageddon, arrived late to the show because her car ran out of gas on the highway. Like the fabled astrologer of old who knew the exact number of stars in the sky, but was stumped when asked, "how many teeth do you have in your head?" Stargazers are often quite naïve about daily events and especially about their own psychological faculties as regards the mechanism of hallucination and faulty perception. Many sightings of UFOs are the result of unsophisticated rural people observing weather balloons, advertising blimps, searchlight reflections on clouds, astronomical oddities (such as Jupiter in conjunction with a full moon), and unusual man-made surveillance devices purposely meant to be "unidentified." Deep-rooted self-deception also plays its part in those cases that seem to be something more than hoaxes or a play for free publicity. These concern individuals who are either calmly fishing at a river or driving home on a lonely, peaceful road when suddenly they are enveloped in a blaze of celestial light. Later they discover that they have lost two or three hours of time. Under hypnosis (a process that seems indispensable to the recall of their experience), they relate all the predictable details of little green men with bulging eyes and whirring antennae. No one has credibly seen or photographed their interplanetary captors, per se. A post-hypnotic view is all we ever get, far less than any respectable spiritualist or ghost chaser usually provides. In the rare cases where "captured-by-spacemen" reports are not stunts or the extrapolations of irresponsible reporters, the psychological problem of hallucination or hypnotic fantasy fulfillment —such as experienced in cases of regressive reincarnation—must be viewed as motivational.

The quasi-fascistic problem earlier discussed, regarding the occult, also surfaces on occasion in connection with UFO-type cults. The most publicized of these is directed by a cryptic couple known simply as Him and Her. The Him has been identified as a former opera singer named Applewhite and the Her as a nurse who took care of him while he was reportedly recovering from a mental breakdown. These two have been recruiting—or in some accounts, snatching—disciples who believe the couple will shortly die and be resurrected in advance of an imminent Doomsday. Some sixty persons, according to the press, have so far disappeared out West, presumably to join this UFO cult. It is their hope, say witnesses, that they will be rescued from Doomsday by UFOs in the control of Him and Her. By the end of 1975, it was reported that some 200 more persons had joined the cult and were now busy proselytizing others to do so. It is widely believed that Him and Her resort to a form of mind control, possibly hypnosis, to persuade followers of their mission.

Carl Sagan, a Harvard astronomer concerned with extraterrestrial probabilities, believes that it is perfectly possible for other humanoid civilizations, like the one on earth, to exist in space, but he points out that alleged sightings of UFOs result "not so much from scientific curiosity as from unfulfilled religious needs. Flying saucers serve, for some," he says, "to replace the gods that science has deposed."[9]

## *Gods from Beyond*

In some cases the "gods" themselves, in the form of space visitors, serve to replace the gods of human credology. These are the creatures who allegedly visited our tiny planet in prebiblical times and who left evidence of themselves in such far-flung places as the Egyptian desert and the Nazca plain of Peru. Erich von Däniken's *Chariots of the Gods?* is the most popular handbook of this notion, although it has been an underground "revelation" for at least twenty years, particularly popular in France. Superficially, the astrogods theory is not really occult or supernatural since it implies the real-life landing by real-life men (at least manlike beings), who either seeded our planet after their own likeness or taught our ancestors the secrets of building unusual monuments, such as Khufu's pyramid at Gizeh (which even so took twenty years to complete). Essentially, this is an euhemeristic notion of theology—the deification of heroes—and occurs in Chinese and South American Indian religions without much dependence on astrogod elaborations. In purely religious, that is euhemeristic terms, the von Däniken idea is no worse or better than speculative interpretations of Genesis (which astrogod worshipers also provide). But when the gods and their chariots turn occult and are called upon to perform miracles and transformations, then the rationalist, and after him the psychologist, must be invoked. A mathematician named Maria Reiche, of Hamburg University, explored the huge carvings of linear figures on the Nazcan plain, which are best seen from the sky and therefore believed by von Däniken and others to be ancient runways or landing fields for the astrogods. Reiche describes them, however, as purely religious (or tribal) decorations carved in homage to the gods—the "real" gods that is (the invisible and theological kind). Small sketches for the Nazcan figures are still visible in fact, she reports, near the mammoth pictures.

Once we can establish the earth-bound origins of much astrogod "evidence," we come face to face with the essentially neurotic, or superstitious, nature of "visitors from outer space." Perhaps the best-remembered large-scale emotional reaction to this cosmic conceit occurred in 1938 when Orson Welles broadcast his version of H. G. Wells's *War of the Worlds* and panicked thousands of casual American radio listeners who took the play to be an actual news report. The so-called sick imagination of many mental patients frequently conjures up "Martians" and space visitors who may be described as elements in a sort of schizophrenic delirium tremens. Persons who are privy to cosmic or visionary information believe themselves specially chosen for their insights and can provide highly developed details parallel to the type sometimes found in schizophrenic fantasies.

A letter I received from a man in Arkansas concerning my views on astrology revealed this sort of disturbed stargazing attitude, replete with fantasy names and dates, as well as highly developed cosmology and a rather ominous antagonism for earthlings.

There were fifteen major inhabited planets in the universe and fifteen minor planets in the universe, the gentleman believed but the "Tantalusians" destroyed the major planet Ceres six thousand years ago, dating backward from "February 14, 1989 A.D.," according to the Gregorian calendar. All mysticism, and this includes all secret artifice, must end, the writer demanded, otherwise individuals who maintain mysticism will lose their "manifest bodies." To be more accurate, "Mankind is Doomed . . . all Fallacy must go!" So individuals had better be preparing for the last and horrible war evidenced by the presence of UFOs.[10]

These angry ravings have the same fundamentalistic Doomsday timbre about them that one finds in the "thick-coming" fancies of Edgar Cayce, the legendary American seer, one of whose specialties was the buried kingdom of Atlantis and its mantic radiation. In 1940, Cayce prophesied that Poseidia, as he called Atlantis, would rise again in 1968 or 1969. Two hundred research geologists and others sponsored by Pepperdine College of Los Angeles in May of 1974 began to investigate the Cayce claim (Atlantis having *not* risen in 1968 or 1969) and covered themselves with ridicule when nothing was found. Was their motivation geological or archaeological, or were they, like most Atlanteans, impelled by Cayce's quasi-biblical fantasies? After all, he had claimed that the "200,000-year-old culture" of Poseidia was somehow affecting life in the United States, which had absorbed Atlantean ideals born out of the war between "the Children of the Law of One" and "the Sons of

Belial."[11] On top of this, the Atlanteans, he reported, created a great solar crystal as a source of energy and rejuvenation that somehow still operates in the area of Bimini, the same general neighborhood as the ominous Bermuda Triangle. Indeed, advocates of a "spooky" theory for why so many ships and planes have allegedly disappeared in that area claim, among other things, the Caycean view of some enormous underwater force (either extraplanetary or Atlantean) drawing these vehicles to their untraceable doom. The fact is, of course, that many of the supposed untraceable and uncanny losses in that particularly turbulent sea are neither uncanny nor untraceable as Lawrence David Kusche reports in his refreshing book *The Bermuda Triangle Mystery:—Solved.*

Dependence on uncanny cosmic events is a form of absolutism that pretends to know all the answers in nature by means of superstitious formulas or systems. Astrology is pre-eminent among such systems and space fantasies provide many of the mantic formulas. The underlying human anxiety that promulgates these attitudes is not to be scorned. The cosmos at best is bewildering and often alarming. However, solving the anxieties born of such conditions by superstitious means can only cause a greater bewilderment, intensified by recourse to sun signs, invisible UFOs, Atlantean energy, and similar cosmic delusions. Those requiring this sort of orientation might better avail themselves of the continuing revelations afforded by the cosmic sciences: astronomy, geology, oceanography, and so forth. There's "magic" enough in those areas to satisfy even the most moon-struck imagination.

CHAPTER 7

# *By Lines and Signs*

He was about eighteen years old and approached me tentatively just before I was to give a campus lecture about the occult.

"What does it mean," he asked, "if you step on a pentagram" (the five-pointed star associated with Satanism)?

I fobbed him off with a playful answer, which I thought befitted the question. But he persisted and told me that he believed illness and bad luck had pursued him ever since the day when in summer camp three years before he had been persuaded to "desecrate" the pentagram by ill-meaning friends.

"What kind of trouble have you had?" I inquired, expecting to hear the usual reports of broken engagements, acne, and unsympathetic teachers.

"I was hospitalized soon after," he told me, "in an institution; seems I developed schizophrenia."

This startling and later verified report left me surprised and all the more burdened with the sorry state of perception in our day. For it seems in the last quarter of the twentieth century that the allegations of parapsychology and the occult (often in tandem) carry more weight and meaning in the average mind than the principles of psychology established in the last one hundred years. Here was a young college student, previously institutionalized for dementia praecox, who could not accurately distinguish the most obvious cause and effect owing to his fundamental superstitious anxiety. The desecrated pentagram had brought on the mental illness, he reasoned, in precisely the same way that many psychics and those who believe in psychicism interpret the cause and effect of premonition, intuition, or other mental activities. It is invariably the supernatural at work, they say, and not the natural workings of the human mind.

Increasingly, we are unreasonably enthralled by apparent *extrasensory* perception, more than by the basic sensory perceptions which we all possess, and in varying degrees, utilize in daily life. There are, after all, among us, for example, those who perceive details with the astuteness of a Sherlock Holmes; others clearly remember their dreams; some can calculate rapidly without an adding machine; others paint pictures or conceive chemical formulas; sensitive mothers pick up signals from their children which they unconsciously process for protective and constructive ends; persons living close together or those prepared by suggestive hypnosis often appear to possess telepathic abilities which are probably more in line with unconscious perceptive insight than with brain-wave interplay. The human mind, after all, is a deep and resourceful cosmos of infinite abilities, a fact which psychology long ago revealed in sober, functional terms. What psychology has failed to describe in any detail, however, are those persons who, because of specific neurotic or monomaniacal needs, distort *ordinary* human functions of the mind, such as those just mentioned, into supposedly paranormal aptitudes. As a result, a class of superstitious types has arisen in the world best described by the title Seers. They are people who either earnestly, or more often deceptively, claim to possess what have been described as psychic powers, meaning supernatural (paranormal) abilities to view the future (precognition), alter natural conditions of gravity and form (psychokinesis), read minds or interpret oracles (clairvoyance or ESP), and so forth. Generally, they function on the order of an updated Merlin the Magician or a Superman and because of their claims, which are rarely challenged or tested, they help promulgate the irrationalism which I believe the pentagram story demonstrates.


## "Mild to Wild"


Those who believe in the magical powers of Seers, and thus secretly envision such powers for themselves, may also be classed as Seers as far as the superstitious formation of ideas is concerned. Such people are only passingly impressed wtih the often meaningful work done by those who are called parapsychologists (the best among them being in fact psychologists without the *para,* or "super" implications). The Seer wants magic, not statistics and testing, and so he is drawn to the superstar Precogs (future-readers) and Psychics of the TV-lecture circuit; those who foretell events concerning Hollywood stars, those who appear to "bend" keys with their minds, pretend to measure emotions by auras and bio feedback, interpret dreams prophetically, calculate magic numbers, assay crystal balls, Ouija boards, Tarot cards, I Ching devices, human palms, tea leaves, coffee grinds, and other such "gypsy" avocations. The underlying need nourishing these superstitious attitudes surrounding parapsychology and psychicism—which even well-meaning psychologists often stimulate—may be traced to man's age-old anxiety about the future—what tomorrow holds. While it is an attitude which bolsters most superstitious ideas (particularly those of the Appeaser category), it is best advanced by Seers, practitioners, and followers, for whom everything and anything provides an omen or augury as to future events and the specific teleology of the universe. As indicated, this category—more than most—subdivides among disparate groups, ranging down the line from "mild to wild."

Class A, the least superstitious, concerns authentic parapsychology, dealing with uses of the mind, sleep, dreams, telepathy and hypnosis, thought control, and altered states of perception. Superstitious formation usually enters this area when the parapsychologist or observer decides to absolutize his findings by declaring them "inexplicable" and therefore, by extension, supernatural—the so-called psi (or unknown) factor. Happily, most scientifically trained people will append the phrase "as yet" to "inexplicable," productively depriving what may be an ordinary human faculty poorly perceived of its more outrageous Superman descriptions. Those parapsychologists, for instance, at the Stanford Research Institute in California (not associated with Stanford University), who imply that the performer Uri Geller produces his "psychic" effects by aid of extraplanetary voices and powers (is it the planet Krypton?), may be classified as Class A Seers of purely superstitious inclinations.

Class B (the quintessential Seer) are those professors of psychicism who claim extraordinary powers of precognition and clairvoyance (or ESP) in all its extensions, but who eschew the testing procedures of parapsychology or psychiatry and psychology and prefer to be witnessed in the arenas of television talk shows and press coverage.

Class C (the common garden-variety Seer descended from Merlin, gypsies, and the traditional snake-oil purveyors), those who deal with magic numbers, oracles, omens, and the like.

The last two categories appeal strongly to the superstitious personality and, as a result, often impose specific harm in terms of outright fraud and misdirection. Investigating the methods and motivations of these last two classes and, above all, applying them to what we know of human psychology (not parapsychology), will be the essential purpose of this chapter. The student suffering from dementia praecox whom I mentioned above, though concerned with the laboratory aspects of ESP, had, not unsurprisingly, spent much of his time, he later reported, pursuing the prophecies of Edgar Cayce and the advice of a local numerologist and reader of I Ching.

## The Lower Classes

Students of thaumaturgy, so-called "real" magic as opposed to the show-business variety (Houdini et al.), like to divide their art into two plateaus: high and low. High magic concerns such metaphysical rigmarole as kabala and alchemy, but low magic encompasses precisely Class C of our present evaluation—the soothsayers and others whose own strong emotional needs to pre-empt the future and nature itself are equally matched by the yearnings of their potential clientele, often middle-aged and older women, usually alone, usually financially comfortable, and often hypochondriacal.

One such lady showed me a flyer that had been handed to her one day in the New York subway. The front of the page was printed with the information: "Crystal Ball Reader—can answer any question, can see into any country . . . I can See and Tell you . . . Is your plane trip safe—I can tell." A name, a box number, and a fee (five dollars) was included. The unusual part of this flyer—dozens of which one can pick up any day in any town—was the handwritten scrawl on its reverse. The woman who had scrawled the message called herself Madame C—a Caribbean, who had sat glowering at my friend for some thirty minutes in the subway car. Her "personal" message was this: "I am a psychic. I see visions, etc. I see you have a small brain tumor here on head (left side, top). It is not too large; you can be operated and saved. But if you wait, you will die. I see needles running down your back. You have blurred vision now . . . I am only telling you. It is your life. Now my job is done."

The effect of this missive on my friend was indeed unsettling and she came to me, knowing I had an interest in the occult, in order to assuage her anxieties. Deep down, like many people, she harbored superstitious beliefs that there are indeed people who can see such hidden information by means of crystal balls or psychic mental powers. I advised the lady, who tended to worry about her health, to ease her mind with a medical checkup and then proceeded to a more conclusive method of debunking the "oracle." Taking the flyer, I went to the phone on my desk, dialed Madame C's number, and urged my friend to pick up an extension in the kitchen nearby. When the seer answered, I affected a southern drawl and spoke anxiously about my "runaway wife, ailing baby, and injured arm." Madame C leaped to the bait; she would give me some immediate and very helpful advice, she said, if I promised to come in for a personal session within three days. This I promised.

"Very well," she intoned. "Your wife has run off with another man and your baby will get better if candles in a church are lit for her" (I never mentioned the sex of my unborn child). "As to the injured arm: how did it happen?" (Odd question for a clairvoyant to ask. Shouldn't she know?) "On the job," I lied. Without a pause, she asserted: "It will soon get infected, but I have a strong potion for it, and I can lay on hands for psychic healing besides."

A few more details were passed and I hung up after promising with a trembling voice to visit the lady's uptown apartment at once. My friend returned from the kitchen, smiling broadly. "What a fake!" she exclaimed. "Who? Me or the Seer?" I chortled. "Both of you, of course. But you've made your point."

Madame C, true to form, had provided a preconceived answer drawn from a stock repertoire of eventualities: runaway wife equals another man, et cetera. The chances are good that the guess will usually fit (except, of course, when the runaway wife is "married" to a bachelor). On top of this—and here's a most glaring and usually unremembered verity in debunking these frauds—if Madame C and her ilk really possessed such powers as she claimed, she could practically rule the world and would surely by now have liberated herself from the drudgery of soliciting five-dollar visits in the subway or receiving clients in a ghetto flat.

## *"Gypsy" Techniques*

But Madame C's claims and techniques, despite their shallowness and sham, are as old as civilization and may even be traced to the prehistoric shamans, rainmakers, and witch doctors (or healers), modern counterparts of whom function today in aboriginal societies and among minority groups in the urban centers. By and large, such clairvoyants, now as the past, require the use of a device which serves, they say, to stimulate their ESP, although inherent magic powers also reside, they claim, in crystal balls, Ouija boards, and the like, by virtue of divine intercession (probably satanic, if anything). Such powers are reinforced by the hypothesis referred to in discussing astrology (the previous chapter), namely, that the macrocosm reveals itself in miniature form via man's own body and natural surroundings. The following practices are supposed to have been passed down by the ancient Egyptians, who wandered through Europe under the nickname "gypsies"—a nickname that only applies in English, I hasten to add. They were, and remain, masters of such divinational systems as reading palms, crystal balls, cards (Tarot and gin rummy), tea leaves, and coffee grinds. From their systems sprang similar divinational antics, such as phrenology (head-bump reading), omenology (reading signs in nature, such as cloud formations), facial forms (blue eyes mean kindness), dream interpretation (not Freudian, rather predictive), brewing and concocting magical potions, salves, charms, and so on.

On a slightly higher plane than gypsy fortunetelling stands numerology, which the Greeks apparently introduced into Europe. There was also a Hebrew form called gematria, practiced in Talmudic times. The Muslim, for his part, introduced the Tarot cards (allegedly conceived by magicians in Morocco, the French for which is Maroc, hence Taroc—or Tarot) and from China comes the mantic practice of I Ching (the Book of Changes).

Ouija boards, as far as I can see, may have originated during the 1920s in the Woolworth "five and dimes."

Common to all these practices is the venerable superstitious idea that such-and-such at point A (a crease in the palm, a cloudy crystal ball) equals or portends such-and-such at Point B (the crease means a stormy marriage, the cloudy crystal a period of doubt). Wordplay and idea association are indispensable to interpreting the lines and signs of low magic. But equally essential is the peculiar idea harbored by all recipients of these ploys that simple or apparent explanations in nature *cannot* possibly be conclusive. If I demonstrate that the hand could not move, even as much as to make a fist, let alone play a piano, without the creases and bumps on the palm (and elsewhere), this does not seem sufficient to explain these peculiar markings. In certain minds they must mean more, even as darkening skies and heavy clouds always mean impending rain. And if anyone doubts the divine aspects of these lines and signs, especially as concerns palmistry, the Holy Book comes along to authenticate the practice in Isaiah 49:16, where it says: "Behold I have graven thee upon the palms of my hands . . ."

## *Numbers*

Though most Seers and their disciples depend on a variety of systems and methods, interchanging Tarot, astrology, and precognition, each system, because of an inherent psychological appeal, beckons a particular superstitious attitude as follows:

Numerology asserts that the digits one to nine are empowered with specific meanings (two, for instance, is a dualistic force) and that one's birth date, plus the numerological rendering of one's name, may be considered a kind of arithmetic horoscope in terms of personality and destiny. The appeal here is to the "scientific" aspect of the superstition, one that is encouraged by recourse to numbers and the Einsteinian powers of math.

Counting, especially of money, is an age-old magical practice—as is naming something formerly unnamed. When King David counted the population of Israel, as earlier reported, God punished him for taking such divine prerogatives unto himself. The farmer counting his crops and harvest feels a sense of power and security in doing so, as anyone does when enumerating his assets. In this regard, all things may be counted or numbered, even a name, a birth, or an address. Though never as popular as astrology, numerology has thousands of followers today, who say that numbers are at least universal factors, unchanging and utterly dependable aspects of truth, which is true when adding, subtracting, or performing similar mathematical procedures. But somehow, science seems to slip away when we learn that the number eleven stands for "success in television or the communications media" or that three is a generative number related to the *three* sexual parts of man—one penis and two testes!

## Palms

Numbers may be universal, but for specificity the Seer will turn to the human palm, no two of which are alike. Because of this rather obvious observation, it follows that specific readings can be had from specific palms; no two readings therefore will be alike. The appeal of personalism or singularity is strong where cheiromancy is concerned and some Seer followers eschew every other magical method in preference for a palms-up perusal. Lines or creases are pre-eminent in this consideration, followed by mounds or bumps, over-all shape, cross hatchings, and whorls. Depth of the life line (the one bordering the ball of the thumb), for instance, implies a deep-meaning life; the mound of Venus relates to love and aesthetics (it is, in fact, the ball of the thumb). A bulging, fleshy specimen speaks for itself.

The unconscious appeal of palmistry is practically universal owing to its specialized quality and gypsy mystique. To test this appeal, just announce at your next cocktail party or at any bar that you are a cheiromancer and behold the sudden burst of upturned palms that greet your claims.

## Cards

After palms, gypsies seem to have popularized card reading or cartomancy, to a high degree (Carmen does a whole scene of it in the opera by Bizet). Practitioners of this divination use the ordinary playing deck and depend on a combination of symbols (clubs, spades, hearts, diamonds) and numerology (three is generative; hearts mean love—a three of hearts implies sexual love). How the cards fall, in what relation they lie one to another (a three of hearts near a jack of spades implies a reckless sexual exploitation), and how many are "read" at any time are the essential elements employed. The Tarot deck is composed of twenty-two picture cards, which are also numbered: Death, on his skeletal horse is card thirteen, ergo the dread of thirteen. There are, in addition, fifty-six symbol cards, which are related to the hearts, clubs, and so forth, in a deck of playing cards. Each picture card is invested with allegoric meaning. Death may signify cessation as well as demise (especially if the card falls upside down when played). The relationship of the cards, one to another, their positions, which layout design is used (the cross, the pyramid, et cetera), are all deemed important in Tarot.

Whether with the ordinary deck or the fanciful Tarot, cartomancy's appeal lies in what might be called a sort of roulette, dumb-luck effect, except, of course, it's not so dumb since all such things are thought to be divinely or magically controlled. Flipping the cards in this wise parallels flipping a coin. The superstitious person depends on and accepts this random activity simply because it is so terribly chancy. In other words, if one wants a question of fate to be resolved ("What shall I do, where shall I go?"), why not rely on fate itself and seek the most quickly performed and least complicated method of divination, to wit: a flip? A sort of crude misology, a disdain for reason, obtains in these cases and it borders on nihilism.

The Chinese I Ching system has something of this same sudden-death appeal. By flipping or dropping yarrow sticks (pennies will do), one learns which diagrams of an elaborate destiny code may apply. The method is not unlike Tarot, in which certain designs stand for certain meanings. The Chin Hexagram (a pattern of horizontal lines), for example, represents advancing or retreating with many obtuse variations thereof. For all its ostensible profundity, the I Ching is a chance-luck method of fortunetelling that appeals to Seers because of its randomness and its fussy detail.


### *General Fortunetelling*


By comparison, crystal balls and the Ouija board are downright mysterious and therefore require "expert" interpretation. A fine crystal glass ball naturally tends to cloud over or give the impression of inward changes, which are due largely to internal light diffusion. These patterns may be "read" the way one reads cloud formations and may also be interpreted a hundred different ways. It's all up to the reader and no two will ever give the same prognosis. In Ouija, the player (usually one of two) moves a planchette, or pointer, by the nervous tension of his finger tips, which are lightly touching the pointer; the lighter the touch, the more static surface tension. As the pointer "magically" moves, words are spelled out via an alphabet printed on the board, or numbers are chosen (related to numerology), or the words *Yes* and *No* are selected in answer to specific questions—and to the unconscious motivation of the fingers on the pointer. Both crystal balls and Ouija boards pertain to a form of illusory kinesis, a microcosmic motion either in the glass or through the pointer. Those who think of life and fate adrift on the sands of time or buoyed by "trifles light as air" may find these games satisfying as a means of future casting. Tea leaves and coffee grinds also depend on the divinity of motion. As they settle at the bottom of the cup, grinds and leaves fall into preordained geometric patterns, which the expert can read quite cleverly. A pyramid-shaped design implies ascent; a circle fulfillment; a speck in a circle equals pregnancy!

## Hidden Signals

All these aspects of fortunetelling depend on two other random, mysterious—one might say antinatural—qualities. The first may be called the factor of poetic logic in which wordplay, symbolic coincidence, and allegory are taken to be demonstrations of divine concern. Nothing is what it appears to be in such a philosophy, whether it be creases in the palm, cracks in the sidewalks, coffee grinds, or the rings left on the table by wineglasses. Each can tell us something about fate if we only relate the cosmos to the detail, the macro to the micro. "All our acts are magical acts,"[1] says Aleister Crowley, the twentieth-century magus. "As above, so below" echos the medievalist from the past. The mystique of believing that "every little movement has a meaning all its own" is powerfully comforting to Seers, who also believe and count on the quaint and charming idea expressed in the Talmud that a man never knows on what day or in which hour his fortunes will change.

If the universe is a plethora of hidden signals, magically or poetically obscured, as the above mystique suggests, then a quick stab or flip at the occultic veil is likely to turn up precisely the right, uncomplicated answer. Since every *thing* is a signal, then every (or any) action taken is sure to hit on the appropriate detail. Chance, synonymous with luck or fortune, in this case implies sudden and, more importantly, accurate knowledge. Such an affection for randomness—like a reliance on poetic logic—is born out of an impatience with the usual rational procedures of thought and decision. Those anxious about the future, about fate in general, come to realize that they are dealing with ineffable, ephemeral forces, which do not easily yield to logical or tedious investigation. How vain it seems to attempt, therefore, a future casting via a computer. The future is too elusive, too abstruse for such calculating devices. Better a lunge, a grab, a flip of a coin or a card.

The problem here is that the chancy evaluation, the "fortune" lightly taken from the context of poetic and ephemeral niceties, is nevertheless viewed after the fact as an ineluctable power, unchanging, fixed, and fated. The formula of this delusion seems to be that a chance action chosen according to a poetic notion invariably produces a conclusive datum concerning one's future and fate. Taken to extremes, one might choose his friends by the following method: Simply select a street with a lucky number (based on numerology), choose an apartment house whose color you believe is similarly lucky (reds, for instance, mean romance), close your eyes, extend your fingers toward the house bell, and ring. Whoever answers is fated to be a significant encounter, at least according to the misology of Seers.

A grab bag of lines and signs of the type so far described would include some of the following common, and probably harmless, superstitious notions, all extrapolated from poetic logic (or illogic, if you prefer). Psychologists sometimes refer to such ideas as "half beliefs"—halfheartedly held, but unconsciously relied upon.

Whistling is bad luck at sea because one might thereby "whistle up" a storm; whistling in a theater dressing room may also be malicious, offsetting proper cues and thus causing confusion. When someone's ears feel hot or are "burning," it implies "warm" sentiments being uttered about the individual, who thus magically "hears" the distant praise. Ringing in the ears, however, implies bad news, such as a tolling bell portends. A sneeze, because of its association with the breath of life (earlier expounded), preceding a statement of opinion signifies that the opinion will come true, since those "returning from the dead" (i.e., sneezing) bear precognition of truth. A pregnant woman frightened by a giraffe may give birth to a long-necked child. And finally, the clavicle bone of a chicken or turkey—the wishbone—answers wishes if one wisher secures the larger piece when breaking it with another wisher. In this, the question remains: Did the name of the bone precede its power, or did the power supply the name?

## Psychicism

The American-Yiddish writer Isaac Bashevis Singer was recently quoted on the subject of faith and psychicism. ". . . It is my conviction," he said, "that telepathy, clairvoyance and premonitions do exist and do have a value. And the more I hear about them, the more comfort I get, because this means that life is just not some soap bubble which today flies around, and tomorrow, in a second, it bursts."[2]

Singer, among other well-meaning intellectuals, as well as persons of lesser mental achievement, has turned for his "comfort" to a new faith in our times: psychicism, the faith of the Seer. They look to this illusory belief aggravated by a basic doubt about life and its soap-bubble effect. This is an understandable doubt, healthy in its intellectual stimulations, but pitiful when it must fall back for buoyance on what is described as telepathy, clairvoyance, and premonitions. In most cases such reliance is based on the flimsiest evidence, and worse, on the performance of well-known Seers that often verges on crass show-business legerdemain. Because the evidence is more a soap bubble than life itself and the psychics, by and large, patent frauds, one must assume that a deep neurotic motivation—one that cannot recognize or cope with reality—supports the kind of comfort Singer and so many others talk about.

Superstitiously, the faith of psychicism is not new. Freud refers to it specifically as "an old religious belief, which, in the course of human evolution, has been pushed into the background by science, or else it represents still another faith, which is even closer to the obsolete convictions of primitives."[3] Every civilized society of the past has had its oracles and seers, many of whom, like the biblical prophets, did not so much prophesy as sermonize—particularly in terms of the prevailing religious or political opinions of the day. The Delphic Oracle in Greece presumably spoke mantic phrases, unintelligible to all but the priests of Apollo, who "interpreted" what she said, probably to their own advantage. The history of psychicism thereafter becomes a parade of glittering superstars, allegedly gifted with precognitive, clairvoyant, and psychokinetic powers: Nostradamus in sixteenth-century France; Cagliostro in eighteenth-century Italy; the Count of St. Germain (a supposed re-incarnate) in the days of Louis XV; David Dunglas Hume, who reportedly levitated in nineteenth-century England; Eusapia Palladino, an oracle from Italy, who was tested and debunked at Harvard University in the early 1900s. All these individuals and many more of our own time, plied their trade surrounded by an aura of legend and reverent anecdote that frustrates conscientious parapsychologists, angers skeptics, and tends to deepen confusion *and* superstition in the uncritical public sector.

## The Case of Edgar Cayce

Edgar Cayce, mentioned in the last chapter in relation to the lost continent of Atlantis, is a prime example of a psychic whose real abilities are lost in an hagiolatry mainly fostered, since his death in 1945, by his sons and the Association for Research and Enlightenment, which they head. This group, in addition to countless books and articles, comprise a veritable industry, alleging Cayce's great healing powers, his abilities to forecast events, to levitate, and to perform other supernormal feats, usually while in a trancelike sleep. What we do know objectively of Cayce is that he was a self-announced illiterate, a deeply religious fundamentalist, and a man fearful that Satan, not God, had provided him with his apparently wondrous gifts—or so it was reported by the New York *Times* in his obituary.

In many ways, Cayce probably saw himself as a later-day Ezekiel (one of his, and all psychics', favorite paragons), and his utterances were faithfully transcribed by worshipful scribes in the manner of the biblical precursor. Early in his psychic career, Cayce—whose forte was always faith healing—built a sort of sanitarium at Virginia Beach, Virginia, a place he believed to possess curative sands.

A hospital and university, based on Cayce's theories, were undertaken at the beach, but went to ruin after the 1929 Crash—an event which, apparently, the Seer had not foreseen. In recent years, these projects have been resumed at Virginia Beach, along with the Research and Enlightenment group. Together, they have become a quasi-religious mecca for Cayceans, who are convinced that their master was the living proof of psychicism as a valid life experience.

Cayce's basic prophecies are generally related to the return of Christ and the betterment of life in the Messianic age. A few mundane specifics also dot the huge body of his so-called telepathic clairvoyant statements or "readings." These include the reappearance of Atlantis in 1968 or 1969; the Christianization of China in the 1950s; the sinking of Japan into the sea; the destruction of cities like San Francisco, Los Angeles, and New York; and several references to unusual scientific and cultural developments that will help solidify Americans against Communism. In toto, however, Cayce's statements, like those of his successors (Jeane Dixon is the best known of these today) are evasive, vague, and homiletic. Speaking in 1933 about whether the United States should recognize the Soviet Union, Cayce predicted: "Many conditions should be considered, were this to be answered correctly. You could say Yes and No, and both be right, with the present attitude of both peoples as a nation, and both be wrong, for there *is* to come, there *will* come, an entire change in the attitude of both nations as powers in the financial and the economic world . . ."[4]

What should strike Seer followers about such statements of precognition or prophecy is not their interpretive truth (after all, there is nothing essentially false about the above evasion), but rather precisely what makes it a prophecy and not simply an opinion such as political columnists express everyday in the press. The batting average of psychics like Cayce who predict the future is unmeasurable when faced by these nonprophecies concerning the inevitable "lessening of tension in the world, or the worsening of conflicts." But when it comes to specifics, the batting average is provably dismal, even below the dumb-luck level of 20 per cent. Jeane Dixon, for example, scores apparently well when predicting natural disasters in the world for any given year (every year, of course, is burdened by its share), but in early August 1974, she stated in print quite specifically that "President Nixon will continue to occupy the White House. He will be found to have committed no impeachable offenses . . ."[5] Within days, Nixon resigned as impeachment loomed. How much safer was Dixon's transparent prediction on the same page that "California Governor Ronald Reagan will be of great service to our country and to the world."[6]

## Occultism in Action

The purpose of this discussion is not to debunk the likes of Mrs. Dixon or the other so-called psychics who parade through the media every day—such as the key-bender, Uri Geller—many of whose demonstrations have been duplicated by show-business magicians. Debunking is a necessary and growing activity where many of these performers are concerned, but of greater importance are the questions that ask: Why do people believe or want to believe the illusory claims set forth in these areas? What motivates the practitioners (besides promises of wealth), and what does it all mean in terms of national mental health? Taking the last point first, one must unhappily again and again conclude that a debilitating gullibility in matters of superstition and the occult is stalking the Western world as it did in the last days of the Roman Empire, and that this disorder does not so much reflect a growing need for beliefs and explanations, which "crass science" cannot provide, as it indicates an extensive psychoneurotic willingness on the public's part to be suckered and eventually tyrannized by all manner of credulity, particularly where psychicism, mind-bending, or downright mystery qua mystery are concerned.

A reporter named Norman Rush, writing in *The Village Voice*, colorfully—but ominously—described an Esalen Institute Conference in San Francisco that had convened to discuss such things as "Using Psychic Powers" and the alleged breakthroughs by the Soviet Union in this direction. One speaker, a political activist named Michael Rossman, presented a rundown of current "far-out" psychic situations that readily serve as a compendium for the heavily neurotic aspects of the subject and also indicate the direction which the anxiety formations are taking these days. As Rush reported it, Rossman began his presentation by waxing enthusiastically over a Soviet psychic who had reportedly killed a frog by remote mind control and then extolled other Soviet psychic experiments which "decondition people so that they can see inside people's bodies and *there is no doubt about it*"[7] (Rush's italics). He further warned that repression of such psychic powers was a capitalistic maneuver. Out-of-body or astral projections, for example, are being countered by "psychic bodyguards" he said, hired to protect people from the occult. Ex-President Nixon employed such bodyguards at the White House.

After discussing other current psychic novelties, such as Uri Geller, Scientology, the giant vegetables grown by psychic forces, and certain aspects of the Hindu-guru trend, the speaker turned to the subject of Elementals. These are, according to the report, "astral entities, not exteriorized portions of our own psyches . . . They confer power. They take various forms. The people who raise colossal vegetables at Findhorn [Scotland] are definitely in touch with them . . ."[8] Seeking control of the world and the future emerged as the resonant purpose of the Elemental revelation.

By itself, this report and the entire Esalen conference may be viewed as an isolated phenomenon. But against the background of increasing concern and experimentation in psychic effects, such as the use of Jimson weed to stimulate the narcotic "visions" of old don Juan, the Mexican Indian dope addict glorified by Carlos Castaneda, or the best-seller status of the shabbily researched *Bermuda Triangle* by Charles Berlitz; against the backdrop of *The Exorcist* syndrome (see Chapter 2), the fascination with reincarnation, oriental out-of-body cults, the tyranny of brain- and thought-modifying organizations, and the general dependence on irrational claims—with all this weighing in the balance, then it seems that Mr. Rossman's Elementals and giant vegetables are no mere oddities or eccentricities, but rather the symptomatic impetigo of public malaise.

In the Middle Ages, sorcerers sought to approach the Godhead through conjurations, Satanism, kabala, and simple defiance of the Church. Marlowe's Dr. Faustus was their paragon. "Seeking control of the world and the future" through the quasi-scientific illusions of psychicism is the war cry of the modern Faustus. In undertaking this campaign, he satisfies a megalomaniacal need in his own unconscious, while radiating the undying fascination of psychedelic, fascistic control over others. (Of course, to the antifascist element, such as Isaac Singer, he offers his mastery disguised as "comfort" in the face of ephemeral life.) In socio-psychological expression, this fascination with psychicism can be seen, in part, as an unconscious concession to parental or religious tyranny, to orthodoxy, fundamentalism, and to certain aspects of spiritual, physical, and mental control, such as if forewarned in science fiction. Seer followers especially want to believe that someone here on earth, a human being like themselves, has managed to grasp the inner secrets of the universe and the mind (thereby) rendering these secrets impotent and exalting man to the status of a god. This is the arrogance and inbuilt spiritual bankruptcy of what Jacob Bronowski calls "absolute knowledge," the sort of thing Hitler professed regarding questions of race, warfare, and morality (as well as astrology). Whereas science perforce admits that it perennially "stands on the edge of error" (again quoting Bronowski),[9] psychicism announces an absolute mastery of enigma through the powers of the enigmas themselves (e.g., the Elementals, remote killing, levitation, telepathy, and so forth). Imagine what power lies within the grasp of the individual who believes he can (authentically) see into the future, read minds, bend metals by brain power, project himself astrally, or exercise the powers of ESP, at least at the gambling casinos—and though no one has come forth who can, in fact, achieve testably true powers through psychicism or accomplish much more than displays of fortuitous guesswork or well-performed feats of legerdemain, the hope remains among those who idolize Seers that the "tricks" of today promise the miracles of tomorrow.

## The Psychological Factor

Two sorts of neurotic tendencies and personalities harbor these basically superstitious (beyond reality) ideas: those who view the world and existence as soap bubbles and who crave comfort from any quarter, no matter how illusive; and those who yearn for the whiplash discipline of tyrants and masters, overblown parents, or gods, who may berate them, incarcerate them (spiritually), enslave them to their strict regimens of control, but who, nevertheless, at the same time liberate them from personal responsibilities, decisions, ponderings, and the gnawings of doubt.

The motivational effects underlying the major tenets of psychicism and the nature of the neuroses and personalities just mentioned can be revealed in the following general outline, which presents the rationales of belief and the inherent dangers of basic psychic superstitions as hypothetically expressed by Seers and their followers:

*Astral effects*—in which out-of-body experiences, including levitation, are thought to occur, and which also encompass such psychic concepts as Elementals and discarnate spirits (poltergeists, or "noisy ghosts," are a favorite in this category).

*Rationale for belief:* "My body is of no real importance or reality. It is ephemeral and therefore something greater must exist, a stronger force, call it the soul, or better, the astral body. I'm glad it exists. My body confuses me, bothers me, reminds me of my mortality and corruptibility—as revealed by Christ. How much better to live a *nonbody* existence here and now, an unpolluted, wondrous condition that raises me quite literally above ordinary men, gives me powers of flight, omniscience, and weightlessness. Out-of-body, I need be burdened by no responsibilities, no shame, no pain at all. I join a universe of elemental forces, become one with God, and immortal while still alive."

*Psychopathological danger* (in extreme cases): dissociation of mental and corporeal functions leading to breakdown of unified consciousness and possible amnesia and/or paralysis.

*Clairvoyant effects*—in which extraordinary mental (telepathic) and sensory powers are manifest with an especial concern for predicting the future and knowing the unkown.

*Rationale for belief:* "Life is an enigma. My existence, my purpose, where I'm going are all soap bubbles likely to break. There are no material signposts, no dependable rules here below. However, by means of ESP, premonition, precognition, and the like, I and others have shown that some of us can and do indeed *know* through extrasensory means. We have seen the afterlife, the future, the inner mind. We are at the right hand of God. Proof positive of our powers is in the fact that the so-called material world ignores us or derides us. Ours are the greatest gifts of history, the unspoken knowledge which the Gnostic sought, which the biblical prophets preached. We are the chosen ministers of the true message. We *see* with superior vision. We shall therefore lead the blind, who only see with their eyes."

*Psychopathological danger* (in extreme cases): acute megalomania and hallucinatory (multimodal) pathology as the unconscious strains to fulfill compelling conscious fantasies.

*Mind-control effects*—psychedelic alterations, including thought and mind (or brain) control, drug-induced visions, and predictive dreams.

*Rationale for belief:* "The mind is a pliable mass in the hands of those who can properly manipulate it and who know its secrets and processes. Science struggles with mechanical devices. We need only our will power, our extraordinary intelligence and sensitivity to effect change and discipline. True, at times, we may resort to material means, such as chemistry, hypnosis, or specific apparatus. But these are simple aids to the over-all power of our inner psi abilities. What we can do for ourselves, we can multiply a thousandfold for those wise enough to avail themselves of our services."

*Psychopathological danger* (in extreme cases): Drug addiction or "hypnotic" enslavement; severe submission, possibly masochistic. Loss of self-criticism and responsibility; antisocial displays, ergo, possible fugue effect (temporary loss of identity).

*Psi effects*—general unspecified "mysteries," particularly those arising out of Soviet research, including psychokinetic movement, Kirlian photography of auras, poltergeists (sources of inexplicable kinetic reactions), eyeless sight, dowsing (the divining rod), table tipping, energy fields, acupuncture, plant bionics (or psychic life), et cetera.

*Rationale for belief:* "Who says life is an enigma or that knowledge is fleeting? We have discovered a secret factor in the universe, the psi factor, which demonstrates that everything can be known or explained and measured, such as the astral body in Kirlian photography. Even gravity is subject to the psi factor and can be suspended by those gifted with the fundamental powers of the universe. We can control material bodies, energy, light, motion, our blood streams, everything we wish, through the untapped powers of phenomenology, which are only phenomena to the ignorant, but which are tangible realities for us."

*Psychopathological dangers* (in severe cases): Absolutism and monomania in which every cause and effect is related to a factor that presumes to explain, but in fact only masks, the inexplicable. Acute delusions may result as every unknown situation is labeled psi without further perusal.

In the above general conclusions, it may be seen that a specific type of psychoneurosis, and possibly psychosis, is likely to emerge from persistent and compulsive immersion in the superstitious aspects of psychicism. Etiologically, the individual tends to formulate his unhealthy belief around some orthodox religious notion (Messiah, post-mortem salvation, reincarnation, spiritism) resulting from childhood rearing or a need for religious identity, which nevertheless resents traditional faith. A strong element of superiority or elitism begins to dominate these attitudes; an ability to hallucinate and a craving for psychedelic experience (usually by use of drugs) is also often apparent. The need for severe discipline and security likewise obtains here as it does with those steeped in cosmic ideas (see Chapter 6). Above all, an anxiety about life, death, and purpose is abnormally strong. The enigma threatens more than it stimulates; consequently, a sense of loss and disdain greets ordinary events, such as coincidence, hallucination, or dreams. Gradual recognition of extraordinary explanations, which psychicism persistently provides, automatically absorbs the anxiety like the proverbial shot (of narcotics) in the arm.

## Parapsychology versus Mysticism

We have spoken naturally of severe situations and extremes. By comparison, most parapsychologists are sober, unemotional practitioners who avoid elitist proclamations or claims of power. J. B. Rhine, the leader of American psychical research since the 1930s, is a respectable example of a self-critical, cautious, and unsensationalistic scientist, and this applies equally to many of his associates. Soviet parapsychologists also seem outwardly unemotional when regarding the alleged powers of PK (psychokinesis), first observed at the so-called Brain Institute of Leningrad, a place I visited in 1970 without succeeding in seeing any firsthand demonstrations of psi or PK effects. I was assured, however, at the time, that neither mysticism nor the supernatural had anything to do with Soviet studies in this area. Gone are the days of the mystic Madame Blavatsky and the Russian occultist George Gurdjieff (a sort of Slavic Aleister Crowley). A few rare psychics themselves seem convinced of possible psychological rather than parapsychological forces at work as regards their alleged "gifts." Mrs. Eileen J. Garrett, late president of the Parapsychology Foundation of New York, was one of the few popular and reputed psychics actually to allow herself to be tested by psychical researchers under laboratory conditions. She spoke candidly of what she considered the "whole, strange, mystifying psychic gift," which would, in her view, benefit by being "snatched out of the darkness of séance rooms and put into the capable, probing hands of science . . ."[10]

The same surely applies to the areas of psychicism as outlined above—astral effects, clairvoyance, and so forth. These are notions which should be more thoroughly studied by psychotherapists, not so much for their "occultic" considerations as for their function in neurotic formation. A deep-seated belief in clairvoyance, I believe, is as revealing in a disturbed individual as symptoms of kleptomania or sexual impotence and frigidity. All bespeak free-floating anxieties and failure of adjustment. In the case of dependence on clairvoyant effects, the tendency to hallucination perceived as precognition (or premonition) might very well reveal itself in psychotherapy.

## Public Airings

The growing power and attractiveness of the psychic mystique likewise represents a faulty *public* perception of general neurotic behavior. What was once commonly evident as megalomania or monomania, as hallucination and dissociation, are more and more passed off as psychic talents of a profound and glamorous dimension, especially on television talk shows. On such airings, phony prophecies made about celebrities, such as Jacqueline Kennedy Onassis (or any Kennedy), about royal families, and political fortunes are never investigated as to fulfillment. Only the lucky guesses are remembered, the frequent bloopers are overlooked. A serious problem is thus created by the media regarding the superstitious "greening" of America (and it is equally true in Europe and Japan), one that demands some scrutiny by the networks and the talk-show people themselves. The saintly, "gifted," holier-than-thou affectation that most psychics display on television should not be allowed to pass for authentic paranormal mental abilities. A little debunking, therefore, before millions cannot hurt in order to put things in proper perspective and hopefully clear the air of the superstitious pollution now heavily upon us.

A word about faith healing in this context is offered, since the subject was raised in reference to Edgar Cayce. Regarded as an element of religion (Christ and Elijah were, after all, healers), faith healing or the laying on of hands, like resurrection, which was previously discussed, need not be superstitiously conceived, that is, regarded as supernatural or magical in effect. This does not suggest approval of its use in lieu of medicine, any more than religious confession precludes psychotherapy. The beneficial effect of spiritual "health" stimulated by spiritual "medicine" is a reality, though it may be short-lived. Individuals enjoying it must be extremely critical of its lasting values and never ignore professional help in tandem with their religious healing. Recent exercises in "psychic surgery," however, which claim to remove tumors or diseased organs without incision (and without leaving scars) are regrettable forms of deceit and legerdemain, often requiring police investigation.

## Letter from a Would-be Seer

Because of my lectures and public appearances discussing the occult and related fields, I frequently receive unusual mail, some of it helpful in understanding the problems of credology and psychology in society today. A letter I received from a lady in Florida, and my reply to it, represent, I feel, a good capsule and summary of the superstitious personality in terms of specific psychic definitions. The letter was rather long and more-or-less catalogued a lifetime of out-of-body, premonitory, and precognitive events, all almost proverbial in character. From me, the writer sought explanations of these "strange experiences," which she had kept to herself for fear of being thought "crazy."

The letter began by recounting an experience that occurred when the writer was "around ten or twelve." She was standing on the pavement with a group of children, and like them, wearing roller skates, when one of the others pushed her and sent her rolling down the driveway, gaining speed as she went. So fast did she roll that she couldn't turn and so went right into the street where two cars were approaching in opposite directions. "A hand took hold of my shoulder," she wrote, guiding her to the right in front of the first car—then up the street between the two cars as they passed each other. She was not at all frightened because that hand was "guiding me . . ."

The second impressive experience that happened to this lady occurred when she was sixteen. Her father had a severe stroke and, as a result, did not recognize her, which, she wrote, nearly broke her heart. A few days later, the writer "saw" her father at the foot of her bed, standing in a strange, soft, golden light. He told her he had come to say good-by. A few minutes later, her aunt informed her that her father had passed away. "I know," the writer responded.

The next experience was even stranger, the lady continued. She was on the operating table, losing a great deal of blood—and suddenly she wasn't there any more, she was in a "perfectly beautiful place . . ." Two children dressed in togas appeared, suffused in the same soft, golden light that she saw in the premonition of her father's death. Then, suddenly, she was back on the operating table and heard the doctor saying: Thank God! Later, he told her and her husband that he had been certain his patient would die, but he hadn't given up, and made one last effort to start her breathing again, hence her return from "paradise." Another, similar, out-of-body effect occured when she gave birth to a stillborn baby and witnessed "from above" the desperate efforts of the physicians to save the child.

Several years later the writer came to the Washington area by bus. The night was extremely hot and muggy and the bus was not air-conditioned, making her drowsy from the heat, but she was not asleep. Suddenly, she "saw" a huge road-repair gravel truck topple over on top of a small compact car. Later, turning on a radio for the news, she heard an announcer saying that an accident had happened nearby, in which a large road-repair truck had turned over on a small car, killing the woman inside. She wrote that she was almost numb at the shock of having "seen" the incident so clearly.

Again in Washington one day, the writer witnessed from the street a motorcade in which President John F. Kennedy was riding, and the thought flashed in her mind that he would die young. She then looked up at a hotel across the street from where she stood and realized how easy it would be to shoot JFK from one of those windows. When she heard the news, some time after, that Kennedy had been shot in Dallas by a sniper she cried and felt that she should have warned him in some way.

The writer then relates a terrible "brooding" she experienced concerning the re-election of Richard Nixon in 1972. She felt so strongly about it that she urged everyone she knew to vote for Alabama's governor, Wallace. About the same time, she had a vision that a congressman reported lost in an airplane crash was in fact alive and wandering in a forest.

She concluded her letter to me remarking on warnings of minor significance, which, if she had heeded, would have saved her from making "mistakes" in her work. Unfortunately, now that she was aware of their value, they did not occur as frequently as when she was younger.[11]

I began my reply by advising the lady that it was extremely difficult to analyze and explain by letter "what appear to be psychic phenomena. It's very much like a doctor giving a diagnosis over the telephone. However, I believe it is possible to apply a certain rule of science to all the things you took the trouble to enumerate in your letter. The rule is this: Never accept a psychic or supernatural explanation for any event so long as a realistic and natural explanation—no matter how farfetched—can be applied.

"I assume that you are a very sensitive person," I continued, "who has suffered from poor health on occasion and from personal tragedy. As such, you are likely to overemphasize natural occurrences, coincidences, or instances of regressive premonition, where you think you sensed something *before* the fact, when actually, the sensation occurred after the event, as in the case of your father's death. There you were impressionably saddened about his illness and pained that he didn't recognize you. Then you learned of his death. Your mind apparently played a common, though imperceptible, trick on you, allowing you one last imaginary visit with your father in a golden glow at the foot of your bed. The same regressive ideation may have occurred that hot summer night on the bus when you overheard, while half asleep, an actual newscast or discussion about the overturned gravel truck. For some reason, this idea provoked a form of trauma in your mind and caused you unconsciously to disguise the news as though it were a precognitive message. You were then alarmed, but mentally prepared, when verification came via the radio where the story was repeated as you had earlier unconsciously heard it.

"In the same vein, many people observing a president riding in an open car wonder about his safety and have unconscious, possibly unpleasant, thoughts about assassination; these they translate into unwilling prophecies. You say on that day of the Kennedy motorcade, you looked up at a nearby hotel and thought how easy it would be to shoot someone from that vantage point. Your mind was clearly dwelling on these possibilities, which unfortunately in the case of John F. Kennedy, were soon to be realized. Common sense and a morbid tendency (which you perhaps rejected by casting it in the form of a 'vision') were responsible for your so-called 'warning' in this case.

"After several years of research and investigation, I must conclude that supernatural occurrences are, in fact, *natural* in origin, either as tricks of the mind or problems of personal neurosis, especially when they involve near death, accident, disaster, or family loss. Few psychics ever get 'premonitions' about delightful and happy events, or ones unrelated to celebrities or their own immediate concerns.

"You say now that you have become more aware of your warnings, they occur less frequently. Perhaps your current awareness is coupled with an innate sense of realization that reasonable explanations are at the root of your apparent 'psychic ability.' Coincidence, daydreams, wish fulfillment, and so forth, no longer impress you as being special or extraordinary things. That's good. Life is complicated enough without anxieties about normal body functions and mental perception.

"It was Francis Bacon, that great rationalist *and* mystic, who noted 'that some minds are stronger and apter to mark the differences in things, others to mark their resemblances . . .'[12] In short, our minds are wonderful and varied. They can perceive red to be green, vapor to be form, and now to be then. But they are not magical entities because of this. Nor are certain people more gifted than others because they perceive the differences more than the resemblances. The real probability is that they are *less* gifted, in fact; less capable of discerning natural phenomena from neurosis, delusion, and self-deceit."

CHAPTER 8

## *Fool's Fire*

So far I have implied a generally negative influence residing in superstitious belief, and I have cautioned against this influence since my experience has led me to believe that habitually irrational workings of the mind are like indelible stains: They do not improve the quality of one's inner "fabric" and if enough of them pile up on each other, they may effectively discolor that fabric and change its appearance entirely.

There are, however—and this, as noted, is axiomatic—certain superstitions, which are, at bottom, healthy symbols of humility and good humor, particularly because they are lightly taken and, when performed, accomplish if not psychic regeneration then at least certain functional and pragmatic benefits. Not walking under ladders, for instance, makes good sense simply in terms of safety. Some few superstitious ideas even enrich the soul or create bonds of communication between strangers; a "God bless you" uttered upon hearing a rather startling sneeze. Several help enlighten us (if we treat them lightly) as to the customs and beliefs of our historical predecessors and may therefore stimulate further study and eventual insights into the fascinating realms of religion, folklore, sociology, mythology, and art. The best of these superstitions—the positive ones—will be highlighted here as the frequently weird, frequently wonderful residue of vanished goblins or ghouls. They will possibly help prepare us for the more intensive analysis to come concerning the formation of the superstitious personality and what makes it tick away like a little time bomb of confusion. By understanding this formation, we may come to appreciate certain significant aspects of personality in general. Besides, the mechanics of making our own private formulas, rituals, auguries, and the way we structure superstition in general, is a virtual lesson in ego development. It should not be overlooked for its remedial benefits in these days of pop psychology and instant insight (both of which are preferable to no psychology and no insight at all).

The all-time favorite superstitions, such as knocking on wood, avoiding black cats, and not breaking mirrors, have already been discussed in appropriate sections of this book. Rabbits' feet, four-leafed clovers, horseshoes, and the number thirteen were also examined. They all seem minimally problematic, although the black cat, related as it is to the fear of witches and devils, stimulates unnecessary Dualist memories, which I have noted to be traumatic, especially against an overly strict religious upbringing. But spilling salt, walking under ladders, and opening umbrellas indoors have certain innocuous charms worth exploring in more detail among others.

## A Grain of Salt

Salt, the great preservative and imparter of flavor, was apparently used by the ancient Egyptians in their elaborate embalming procedures. Besides, because the great womb of life, the sea, was salty to the taste, man from the first associated sodium chloride with life (the after*life*, included). Roman soldiers received a portion of salt (or the money to buy it) as their salary, their word for which (*salarium*) meant "pertaining to salt." Witches scorned the life-preserving reputation of the tasty crystals and spread the rumor that spilling salt meant forsaking life, or at least inviting a bout of misfortune. Da Vinci in his mural *The Last Supper* has taken this notion to heart. An overturned container of salt may be seen in front of the treacherous Judas, who sits to the right of Christ.

As witches tossed water over their left shoulders in order to raise storms, so it became propitiatory to pinch up a bit of any salt that had spilled and do as the witches thus "raising" again one's fortunes and life and, at the same time, tossing "life" (in the form of salt) in the invisible faces of the demons and fiends who ever lurk at the left hand of man (the "sinister" hand). Though this may be a somewhat messy ritual (salt underfoot affords a distinctly gritty sensation), it nevertheless reflects commendable values and respect, first for the salt itself—which in its day was a fairly precious commodity —and then for life itself, a concept always worth its share of reverence.


## Ladder phobia and Threes

Reverence is the basis of the ladder superstition, but, as noted, sensible precaution may have also been the pragmatic motivation for avoiding sallies under ladders leaning precariously against walls. One may overturn a ladder while walking under it, or something may fall from it onto the head of the walker below. More important to the superstitious person is the fact that the devil allegedly lurks at ladders, as he did near the one used to raise the Cross on Calvary. In the same vein, a ladder leaning against a wall forms a triangle, or trinity, through which one should not walk in respect for the Father, the Son, and the Holy Spirit. A reverence, or fear, of the number three implied by this superstition, is the basis for similar considerations. We don't light three cigarettes with one match, lest Satan see the flame and snatch the last recipient (or enemy troops do the same for soldiers in the trenches of World War I). Three can be lucky, of course—again the Trinity concept is at work. Repeated efforts are often rewarded the third time around; fairy tales consistently show us that the hero must attempt some difficult ordeal at least three times—on the third attempt he will succeed. Three riddles, three guesses, are similarly proposed in both legend and life. It is the endless procession of fortuitous (or if badly treated, malignant) trinities that informs this idea—trinities of religion, mythology, the deepest recesses of the human mind, and the most common practices of daily life: Father, Son, and Holy Spirit; Abraham, Isaac, and Jacob; Zeus, Poseidon, and Hades, (sky, sea, and earth); Brahma, Vishnu, and Shiva (in India); superego, ego, and id: Tinker, Evers, and Chance (three strikes, you're out!).

In a sense, opening an umbrella indoors relates to traversing the trinity (walking under a ladder), since it seems to imply that one is thus defying the natural use and order of things by opening in the house an object clearly intended for outside. Oriental chieftains regarded the umbrella, or parasol, as sacred, and the more numerous such coverings held over their heads, the more esteemed and sacred they could be deemed. The pagoda in India, an architectural form that spread throughout the Buddhist world, was originally a shrine composed of several pyramiding parasols, connotative of sacred respect for Buddha himself. To belittle such a symbol by carrying it open under a roof seemed sacilegious. It is also a clumsy thing to do since one may flip open an umbrella in the living room and knock over all the bric-a-brac. Besides, who needs a reminder indoors of rain?

Likewise one does not, or should not, toss his hat on a bed. As a covering for man's sacred seat of wisdom (his head), the hat was regarded as symbolic of status and reverence, possibly for life itself. It should not, therefore, be associated with sleep or death (humans often die in bed). Anyway, a nicely formed fedora plunked on a bed may be sat upon and crushed, so there is here, as with most beneficent superstitions, a secondary practical consideration to observe.


## The Hallowed House


Rooms, doors, numbers, all interplay in the superstitious formation, just as the natural, or sacred, order of things may be observed in the ladder-umbrella-hat canards. In Great Britain, one never sweeps dust and dirt out of the living room or main-hall door of the house, lest you sweep out life and luck as well. One must gather up the debris and deposit it in a container or maneuver it to the back door, where it belongs. The idea originates with a reverence for thresholds, imparted by the Romans, who kept a special servant stationed at the front door to help lift a visitor's foot over the threshold, thus preventing desecration. (Such servants were known as "footmen.")

If three is sacred, apartment dwellers should probably like to live on the third floor of a house; certainly not on the thirteenth (few do these days since obliging landlords usually skip the ominous thirteenth story, which they call *fourteen*). But no matter what floor a person lives on, it is supposedly bad luck to move downward in the same building for fear he might lower his fortune as he approaches the ground (as ever, wordplay is at work in superstitious ideas). A man I know was so disturbed when his daughter moved from the sixth floor to the fourth that he sought "professional" help and learned from an indulgent rabbi that misfortune could be averted if the movers brought a single chair from the sixth-floor apartment to the street before occupying the fourth-floor flat. Also, the rabbi added, "tell them to leave the sixth-floor door open when they have removed everything from the premises."

Such rituals appease the mind, and more significantly, memorialize the big event of moving, thus causing certain unconscious ambitions of success (or luck) to be doubly exerted in the new surroundings.

For something of the same reason, certain people will switch chairs at the dining room table or at their desks, or turn armchairs now facing the door to face the windows instead. All this is done in a sort of sympathetic magical manner, a homeopathic twist, in the hopes that new directions of chairs or furniture in general will stimulate new directions of luck. As noted repeatedly, such dependence on word or idea associations is essential to the formation of superstitions and, as we shall see, is an almost instinctive mechanism of the superstitious mind. Because of such things, new clothes will equal new opportunities, especially around holidays (ergo the new Easter bonnet), a journey begun with the right foot will be "right" or good, as opposed to sinister (the word sinister in Latin means "left"). The last rose of summer somehow possesses all the beauty and happiness of the vanished season, but the last bit of food left on the serving tray may impart to the glutton who snatches it up that he (or especially she) will also be last, particularly at the marriage altar. The "old maid" status will also be the fate of those "who are the last ones in"—presumably, in the temple. A lady who finds herself in this predicament (unwed or unwanted) may maneuver herself into a position for catching the bouquet tossed by a bride. If she catches it, marriage for her cannot be far behind, at least Roman virgins who caught such flowers tossed at the marriage god, Hymen, were presumed divinely selected for wedlock and lucky besides.


## Wedding Cakes

If the unwed lady fails to catch the bouquet, she may secure herself a tiny bit of the wedding cake to place under her pillow (the cake is, of course, well wrapped). This is done in the hopes that the fertility symbol, which cake implies, will somehow rub off on the sleeper. In ancient times, all cakes were thought sacred, especially when shaped in human or phallic form (we retain this idea in the bridal figures plunked on wedding cakes). Hot-cross buns are a pagan derivative, adopted by Christianity, of primitive fertility cakes made in the form of an outstretched man. Eating such objects, though they imply symbolic cannibalism, was fortuitous, considering the luck imparted. Tossing rice, and by extension, confetti —or "sweets"—at bridal couples is part of the same fertility ritual. Actually, ancient peoples gave seed and rice to newlyweds to start them on their way toward good crops, good luck, and a well-stocked granary. Shoes, no less precious than seed, could also be given (or tossed) to newlyweds and these days may be tied to the rear bumper of the honeymooners' car in deference to the biblical custom of handing over a shoe as a sign of contract—such as occurs in connection with the marriage of Ruth and Boaz in the biblical Book of Ruth.


### Good Luck—Bad Luck

The word luck, or lucky, has appeared frequently in tandem with the type of superstitions now under consideration. In fact, luck or the lack of it is the basis of most propitiatory rituals and private auguries. There is a deep-rooted and universal notion in human psychology that hovering somewhere in space is this thing called "luck" that may descend at any moment, usually without warning, and change our lives (the winning lottery ticket, the chance meeting of an influential friend, the finding of something precious underfoot). Few people remember that, in fact, what seems to be luck is really the result of conscious or possibly unconscious effort on the individual's own part. The actress who gets her "lucky" break by going on unexpectedly for an ailing star and who thus wins fame and fortune must surely know that without training, talent, and preparation she could have just as easily ruined her career by the seemingly fortuitous event. How many unwon lottery tickets must be strewn about one's floor before the "lucky" one appears? Of course, there is always that one lucky "dog" who buys his first lottery ticket and, behold, it is the winning number. This seems to be proof of something called "beginner's luck" (first things are always blessed, et cetera). But, in fact, it is more likely the dynamics of averages at work. Surely for all those millions who consistently buy losing tickets, there is bound to be one whose first purchase is a winner, just as, during the famous blackout that blanketed the East Coast in 1965, there were bound to be several thousand luck*less* individuals who had just stepped into a moving elevator as the electricity failed.

Luck, good luck that is, will always seem magically won and consequently, over the years many devices, practices, and superstitions, per se, have developed to stimulate or beckon the apparently mysterious *coup de chance*. Occultists revel in this area and have catalogued countless lucky colors, days, numbers, objects, flowers, and so forth, on the theory that "we must assist luck" or guide it. Well and good, so long as we continue to prepare, to reason, to take the proper steps and precautions. *Audaces fortuna juvat*, the Romans said: "Luck does not favor hesitation"—precisely the point. One is "lucky" because one is daring or exertive, not because he sits back in his lucky shirt, on lucky Tuesday, dangling his lucky rabbit's foot or four-leafed clover in a torpor of ineptitude.

For purposes of stimulating one's innate abilities, and as positive spurs to action, the following "lucky" ploys may be of use. One should note that different concepts apply to different dimensions or directions of luck. The formation of these conceits in terms of wordplay, ideologic associations, and variations of sympathetic magic should be, by now, quite obvious, if not transparent.

To achieve luck in love, say the augurs, activities should be undertaken on Mondays, ruled by the romantic moon, or on Fridays, named for Frigga, the Nordic goddess, who presides over marriage (a sort of Teutonic Venus). At such times, apparel of a red, pink, or earthy color favors the passions one seeks. So do red roses and the number six (Venus's number). Business or financial luck may be forthcoming on Tuesdays (named for Tiu, the Teutonic war god). Tuesday is also supposed to be the second day of creation, upon which God, in Genesis, uttered the word *"tov"* or "good" twice, the only time he did so. Thursday is also a day to strike while the iron is hot, as did Thor, the Nordic god of thunder who carried a hammer and for whom the day is named. Colors of gold and silver are obviously fortuitous concerning financial destiny and one may try for those important business conferences or "big deals" around three o'clock (the lucky three) in a room decorated with pink carnations, which the Arabs say is a flower that signals "favorable answers." Believers in such arrangements may indeed experience the fortune they seek, not because of the carnations of the day but as a result of the positiveness these auguries stimulate.

For simple luck of a general variety, efforts undertaken on Saturday favor Saturn, god of planting. In the Roman age, Saturday was sacred (as it is among the Jews); even criminals could not be punished on that day in Rome—lucky for them.

Other fatidic (or magical) considerations of occult persuasion tell us that a gift of gloves is lucky; turquoise imparts success; a found penny auspicious (any found money must be so deemed); bumping into a humpback is fortuitous; being victimized by bird droppings or stepping into manure, excellent luck (what else good can you say about such events?). To upset a box of matches, drop an egg (thereby freeing fertility), find a ladybug (but dare not kill it), all portend luck, change, success—what have you.

Alas, for most superstitiously inclined persons, it is not so much good luck as it is fate, or bad luck, that weighs in the world. Naturally, the *coup de chance* is always welcomed, but more often, say the believers, one must work his magic not so much to stimulate fortune as to avoid the strictures of fate. In this capricious universe, luck deals only with minimal factors, such as the gambler's toss of dice. But fate is the force that may topple kings. It is this fatalistic aspect of luck that tends to traumatize the superstitious mind; a lucky hand of cards, a found penny, and the like will be passed off as inconsequential compared to an unexpected rainstorm on a day set aside for golf or a garden party. This is regarded as bad luck, ill fate, possibly the results of a curse.


## Luck and Health


Few areas are of graver concern in terms of fate or ill luck than is health and, accordingly, numerous superstitions have arisen to protect those who regard illness as an arbitrary, malicious stroke of fate. Arbitrariness, they say, is the cause of disease, therefore, similarly arbitrary, that is irrational or unscientific remedies, should be invoked as protection.

So it is that New Englanders will carry around a gall from the goldenrod or a gnarled knot of a tree as protection against rheumatism. The gnarled or bitter aspect of the charm somehow forestalls similar problems in the body. Many people associate opals with disease and death and eschew wearing these ornamental gems. It is believed this superstition arose during the Crimean War. British soldiers discovered the fiery stone in the area, where it is common, and bought hundreds of opal rings as souvenirs. After the fatal charge of the Light Brigade at Balaklava, it was noted by the burial squads that almost all the casualties bore the ominous opal on their fingers. Was it the cause of the disaster? *The Encyclopedia of Occult Sciences* regards the very same opal as a symbol of "confidence" and tender love.

The French have developed numerous magical antidotes for disease, including drinking an admixture of red wine and melted tallow for sore throats and colds. Predictably wine serves as a basis for many folkloric remedies in France, and elsewhere, as does grease or animal fat. Chicken fat rubbed on red flannel and wrapped around the throat is a Middle-European remedy for tonsillitis. Waving burning chicken feathers in front of children with stuffy noses is supposed to help clear their heads (or else try some chicken soup). Spanish grandmothers brush a child's face with a pine bough also to insure health and growth (or evergreenness).

## Of Clime and Kine

Rustic people regard sudden or ill-timed changes in weather as ominous, not simply because a rainstorm might ruin a golfing date but because of the damage possibly done to crops and livestock. An age-old search for magical indications of climatic fate remains in the superstitions of our day, some of them based on sound empirical observations. A gray or greenish lowering sunset, farmers correctly relate, indicates rain. A patch of blue seen through even the most obstinate clouds promises fair weather and a halo around the moon warns of moist heat.

Less dependable weather signs concern unexpected visits by robins in one's parlor, presaging frost and snow, or the almanac casuistry that says hail in February is a sign of a good autumn to come. Then there is the popular notion about the groundhog, or woodchuck, who, if he sees his shadow on February 2, is supposed to return to his burrow to wait out another six weeks of winter's cold. Oddly enough, this folk belief seems to imply that sunshine on Candlemas Day (which is February 2, a pagan feast) rather than being welcomed, instead portends lingering cold and unpleasantness. Is this because witches, who convened their Sabbat on Candlemas, despised the sun?

While on the subject of animals, three should be mentioned that are involved one way or another with luck; this time happy luck. In Europe the stork is considered a generally lucky bird, one that only nests on sturdy roofs and whose very name, adapted from Greek, means "strength in affection." What better creature to bear babies from the distant marshes of Egypt, where the souls of unborn children allegedly reside? The cuckoo is another fortunate feathered friend, who is supposed to favor propitious time; hence its use in cuckoo clocks. Its distinctive call, when heard in spring, supposedly signals good luck, and Germanic people, upon hearing the first cuckoo, slap their wallets or purses to ensure financial bounty—an act that may unconsciously inspire clever investments in the coming season.

The fish as a cryptic symbol for Christ and an archetype of sea life has long held a special place in the lexicon of luck. Besides being a "brain food," it is said to impart holiness as a substitute for meat (as it once did among Roman Catholics on Friday—a memory of the association of fish with Venus, whose day Friday was in Rome). And then again, every man hopes to catch a fish with a gold piece in its mouth as did St. Peter at Christ's instruction.

Numerous pages could be written on related or extrapolated superstitious beliefs that fulfill the weird and wonderful designation of this chapter, as opposed to the more traumatic effects earlier described. Such pages would teem with imaginary creatures: dragons, unicorns, trolls, sprites, and genii, and they would relate the deep unconscious symbols and prototypes of myth. The manifold meanings, functions, and artistic influences of such imaginary beliefs have been well defined and artfully related to daily life and human psychology by scholars like Jung, Robert Graves, Joseph Campbell, and others. Even more penetrating, however, and possibly more revealing—though less well investigated—is a knowledge of the formation or inception of superstition in the human mind. How and why it begins, as opposed to how it shows itself, and what it demonstrates are the considerations we shall now pursue in discussing the superstitious personality, a bit of which dwells in all of us and goes far to explain current—and past—fascinations with the occult, the bizarre, the irrational—in a phrase, with the *ignis fatuus*, or fool's fire, earlier invoked.


## Searching the Fox


Two of the favorite epithets of the New Testament concern a certain hateful "fox" (Luke 13:32)—who is probably King Herod—and a terrifying beast described in Revelation, Chapter 13, of whom it was written "his number shall be 666." Both Herod the fox and the Beast 666 (who some say was also Herod) are deemed to be the ultimate anti-Christs and as such have been and remain among the favorite fantasies of the superstitious mind. The British magus Aleister Crowley, in the 1930s, discovered that he himself, was Mr. 666, and in St. Louis, Missouri, a few years back, a disabled gentleman "on a fixed income," began writing a series of letters to the Pope, several cardinals, Billy Graham—and *me*, describing his apparently fruitful tracking of the fox and of Beast 666 in one. Both the writer's method and his conclusions demonstrate the unusual workings of the superstitious personality and may help uncover its motivations and formation.

To begin with, Mr. Morrow (as I will call him) declared himself firmly opposed to the practices of witchcraft, sorcery, and spiritualism, although he clearly accepted their magical powers and in fact, as we will see, eventually related the Beast 666 to spiritualism, per se. This apparently dichotomous or ambiguous attitude about "black magic" is often a feature of superstitious neurosis and even religious belief (see Chapter 2). In well-typed, fairly literate form, Morrow then outlined a three-year search that finally identified the beast by means of "theoretical exercises in mental gymnastics," the first of which occurred when he perceived the fact that the fox referred to above is initially mentioned in Luke *13* and that Beast 666 dominates Chapter *13* of Revelation. This uncanny coincidence (although there are no such things as coincidences in the superstitious ideology), coupled with the ominous number thirteen itself, is formidable prima-facie evidence that somehow led Morrow to the next discovery, namely, that the letters F-O-X fall directly beneath the number six, if one assigns numeric values to the alphabet by writing out one through nine in a single row and then filling in three rows of consecutive letters directly below each number.

"Thus," he wrote, "FOX fully satisfies numeric and named requirements . . ." But who is this fox in actuality? Further intensive reading in the biblical text led Morrow to realize that an aspect of this beast (fox) will be its "false prophecy function," stemming from "seeking the truth from the dead." In an "inspired" leap, the researcher then arrived at the news that Fox is the surname of the sisters who, in the 1840s, first systematized spiritualism, "allegedly establishing direct contacts with spirits of the dead." Having gone this far, it now became Morrow's mission to uncover specific evidence of the fox-beast relationship in the modern world and so "last fall, as a last resort" he wrote, letters were mailed "to ALL residences named FOX (approximately 170) in St. Louis Telephone Book. Visible manifestation," he continued: "one visit from one drunken man named Fox, threatening a suit of slander."[1]

Mr. Morrow's "mental gymnastics," as he himself calls them, are, of course, equated by him with the very essence of sensible intellectuality. Unfortunately, the twists and turns of his mental regimen, born of dogmatic conceits and personal anxiety-frustration, quite often produce the kind of actions most ordinary people would describe as "crazy." In such actions, qualitative forms of reasoning manage to emerge along with momentary flashes of insight, so that gibberish or incoherency are not usually the stylistic trappings of the haunted mind when dealing with cosmic considerations. Even so, few of us will ever appreciate either the insights or the style of such thinking when confronted by the inevitably bizarre and often comical results this type of mental gymnastics so frequently provide. The information about the 170 residences of St. Louis named Fox and the "one drunken man" who responded with threats is a perfect example of this sort, proving that it is the functional failure of Mr. Morrow's search, one should say the *inevitably* functional failure, not its style, which, alas, must characterize the entire effort.

Above all, Morrow's search and its finale are conclusively symptomatic of what the psychologist Morton Prince called "the sum total of all the biological innate dispositions, impulses, tendencies, appetites, and instincts of the individual, and the acquired dispositions and tendencies—acquired by experience."[2] In short, he speaks of personality.

Let us draw up a hypothetical case (it could be Mr. Morrow) of the fairly typical superstitious personality by examining the components discussed in Prince's definition and how they may be personalized in the categories we have previously outlined, to wit: Appeaser, Expiator, Conjuror—and so forth.

Almost invariably, the superstitious character evolves from a deeply dogmatic family setting, usually strict religious in belief and practice. In the West, such a family is often—but not exclusively by any means—Roman Catholic or fundamentalist (some say, evangelical). Mr. Morrow, it should be noted, reveals that he is a Catholic. Crowley (Beast 666) was the son of devout fundamentalists of a sect in Britain called the Plymouth Brethren. There have been, in addition, Conjurors from the ranks of Orthodox Judaism and Seers from High Episcopal homes. However, I doubt one would find a truly discernible superstitious personality emerging from a humanistic or genuinely agnostic background unless it was in reverse rebellion to the liberalism which such thinking fosters. A strict religious upbringing is a formidable factor in personality development of any sort. When it is coupled with a literal emphasis on the Bible, particularly on its "magical" passages—the stories of miracles and witchcraft—an intellectual procedure may be established which relates even the most ordinary human proclivities and happenings to wondrous intercessions by God. As soon as the growing child discovers that certain magicians or sorcerers also ascribe to themselves the powers of deity, the chance exists that the formerly religious fascination with miracles may be converted to a superstitious tendency regarding magic, per se. Factors of influence at this point may be the child's exposure to well-developed superstitious personalities; a mother who declares herself to be "a witch" will be bound to influence a religiously haunted child (especially if the child is a girl). Intensive interest in fairy tales, myths, and science-fiction literature, either as read or seen in movies or on television will help convert the respectable and obligatory religious attitude into a more secretive, self-interpreted, or fantasized schema. The child may reason: "Mom and Dad want me to be deeply religious as they are and I want to live up to their ideal. But the sermons bore me and I don't understand the rituals. What I do like are the stories of raising the dead and the witch of Endor and Elijah's fiery chariot. On TV I saw something about UFOs that reminded me of the fiery chariot and I guess the witch of Endor is sort of like the witch in Snow White. If I think of the Bible as a very special book of fairy tales, then it becomes all the more meaningful to me and I become a dutiful child, respectful of my parents' traditions and deserving of love."

Naturally, the mechanism just described does not always lead to full-blown superstitious attitudes. Certain other "mental gymnastics"—to quote the fox-hunting Mr. Morrow—must be additionally present. These pre-eminently include a fascination with coincidence bordering on mysticism. Superstitious people take unexpected parallel events or words as signs of divine intervention and do not realize, as Isaac Asimov points out, that "having no unusual coincidence is far more unusual than any coincidence could possibly be."[3] Similarly appealing and seducing are fantasy images and the very essence of *idea*, i.e., the building of thought upon thought in a self-startling or stimulating manner relative, in some, to a libidinous awakening, in addition to those stimuli which range from purely physical to purely intellectual in form.

We also live our lives of secret and private stimuli in the midst of family and social tensions that, on the one hand, may enhance, broaden, and refine our perceptions or pervert, distort, and cripple them, on the other. Sixteen-year-old Adolf Hitler, when he first heard Wagner's opera *Rienzi*, reportedly raced from the opera house ablaze with imperious ambition, determined to found a dynasty of his own like that of the Roman proto-fascist whom Wagner had immortalized in music. It is said that Hitler, that same night, designed the chief banners, insignias, and uniforms that were later to horrify the world during the Nazi scourge. Conversely, the artist Gordon Craig, the son of Ellen Terry, upon hearing his first Wagnerian opera, set about to design radiant stage settings that have transformed the art of theatrical decor.

The operative factors in perverting (or perfecting) the stimulated attitude are frequently found in parental reaction, sexual security, and a hundred-and-one influences that drift along in the background of a young person's life, imperceptible but highly causal in effect. A child exposed to continuous parental bickerings and disorder, for instance, tends to differentiate even positive stimuli in a protective, anxious manner. Such a child, inspired by the legends of Ovid, for instance, might wish himself empowered with the magic of metamorphosis either to transform himself into a form unrelated to the parental scene or possibly to wave a magic wand over his obstreperous mother and father, replacing them with voiceless doves.

Other problems of differentiation, and integration, may evolve after prolonged traumatic experiences of rejection, sexual confusion or guilt, physical abuse, ridicule, victimization as regards work procedures and other household regimens, and the general slings and arrows to which most of us are exposed. Some psychologists include among these certain socio-biologic strains which chemically or genetically flavor our lives. These, faced with intensive religious (or in some cases specifically superstitious) attitudes, will tend to transform imaginative and sensitive childhood yearnings into blatant irrationalism that becomes, for the traumatized child, the only "rational" means of self-protection and preservation.

## Easy Magic

Our hypothetical case study now passes from childhood to the teen-age labyrinth where confusion, doubt, and enigma are standard decorations, especially as concerns the cosmic questions of life, death, God, salvation, and the supernatural. Because he has been trained to believe fundamental or literal biblical references to angels, demons, and so forth, the incipiently superstitious teen-ager sees no reason why he should not overintegrate these ideas in specifically occultic terms. He will thus proceed to a habitual practice of archaic reasoning and distorted teleology. In this practice, coincidence becomes a form of divine telepathy (exclusively his), ordinary objects take on the nature of omens and symbols of divinity (or deviltry), such as imagined facial shapes in wallpaper patterns or light reflections. Natural enigmas of this sort can only be subdued or understood via magical rites that begin to dominate daily routine, from the invoking of specific incantations (such as mantras) to the avoidance of stepping on cracks in the sidewalk lest they open up to reveal the pits of hell. Even physical factors, one's body, one's sex drive, coloring, handprints, et cetera, are regarded in magical (therefore neurotic) terms.

As the teen-ager grows into adulthood, either one of two degrees of this "easy magic" formularization will have firmly established itself, to wit: the "mild to wild" distinctions I have mentioned before. In the milder cases, a concern for superstitious systems, such as astrology, palmistry, omens, and prophecies may suffice to compensate traumatic conditioning and eventually pacify—but also neutralize—the individual, who usually degenerates into the passive pawn of whatever magical power he believes dominant in his life. The wilder case, unable to appease a burning frustration and ambition, in which world recognition and transformation are envisioned, turns to the "theological" dispositions inherent in his character since childhood. He now converts these into agonizing, possibly violent, aspects of megalomania and psychosis.

## *The Case of Professor Rose*

A common development in the wilder process is for the individual, who has formerly flirted with witchcraft or demonology or psychic phenomena, to declare himself now no longer the apparent being we all perceive, but rather some astral superhuman transformation to which others must eventually bow. In this manner, Charles Manson became a schizoid Jesus-Satan amalgam; Crowley emerged (somewhat less wildly) as Beast 666; the sex-bomb Joanie discussed in Chapter 4, became Scintilla, the witch, and a former university professor I knew in Boston became "I Am," the Jewish Messiah!

Excerpts from this particular individual's literature, which he handed out freely in the streets, are useful in further revealing the mental gymnastics or convolutions consistent with the conditioned differentiation of an intensely superstitious mind. Professor Rose, as I shall call him, is awash in a sea of numerologic magic, which he has probably integrated from childhood exposure to Orthodox Judaism, in which gematria—a sort of kabalistic numerology—plays its part. By gematria, so say the practitioners, whole sections of the Bible may be decoded (numerically) and then reinterpreted as God intended his words to be really understood. Where magic and superstition are concerned, things are never as they appear—even in the Bible. Consequently, mental gymnastics are a *sine qua non* for those who wish divinely ordained power. Unfortunately, because of childhood weaknesses and anxieties, such persons frequently overstrain themselves in their exercises, until certain mental sinews and muscles either warp or snap, as the case may be. Professor Rose noisily parades the streets, red of face, bristling with belligerence and receptive to neither criticism nor compliment as he spouts a garbled biblical text and a plethora of numerical intricacies that would boggle even Newton's intellect.

His own role as the modern-day Messiah is unassailable (he offers a cash prize to those who can disprove it!), since it derives from secret messages of God buried gematria-wise in the names of the first three presidents of the United States: Washington, Adams, and Jefferson. The professor explains:

". . . In the name Adams [is] the idea of the Hebrew word *adam* meaning *mankind*. [Also] . . . the idea of Jeffer *son* and the idea of the concept THE SON OF MAN. Now see the POETIC STATE-MENT in NAMES of the 1st, 2nd, 3rd presidents. The names— WASH ING TON—ADAM S—JEFFER SON. The name WASH-ING TON contains two ideas. The word *washing* is obvious (i.e., to cleanse), the word TON is associated with the idea of 2,000 pounds.

"Therefore—THE POETIC STATEMENT in shaping the names of the 1st, 2nd, 3rd presidents as Washington, Adams, Jefferson is this: THE WASHING OF MANKIND (i.e., washing-adam) BY THE SON OF MAN (i.e., Adams-Jefferson) [will occur] BEFORE THE YEAR 2000 . . . I say to you, He who writes these words to you, is that same MESSIAH of the line of David, I AM THAT I AM . . ."[4] (ergo, the "cleanser" of Man).

An exquisite, almost typical process of rationalization employed in superstitious ideology is contained above. It in no way means to be flippant or cute, but it is intensely perceived and energetically believed. As such, it is identical to the ideological gymnastics of astrology (Mars, the war god, causes belligerency in men), or Satanism (the serpent in Eden was the devil and offered knowledge of sexual pleasure to Eve, therefore, Satan, not God, is the benefactor of humankind), or certain aspects of psychicism (since man has a soul, it follows that the soul may have a life of its own revealed as an astral body).

Admittedly, these tortuous lucubrations seem not unlike certain respectable principles of philosophy or science, logic or theology, since on first glance they all have a superficial consanguinity. This illusory relationship stems from the fact that the occultist is often learned in philosophic and even scientific cant, specifically in its literary style. But the slightest probing reveals several essential and conclusive differences between, let us say, the journal of an astronomer and an astrologer's chart. For one thing, in sensible tracts commonplace elements of coincidence, semantics, facile inference, and hyperbole are ignored or avoided since they more often than not tend to disrupt and confuse any rational issues. If I attempt to prove, for example, that gypsies descended from ancient Egyptians because the letters *gyp* are identical in both generic words, I have only reduced my argument to nonsense by forgetting that in other languages the semantic relationship is nil. Critics, who may have considered the *gypsy* equals *Egyptian* theory on purely historical grounds, now laughingly reject it out-of-hand as a result of simplistic evidence. Indeed, the simplistic seduction of Professor Rose by the nomenclature of Washington, Adams, and Jefferson is prima-facie indication of his faulty "proof" and at once divorces it from serious consideration by serious men. They know that the superstitious mind will invariably probe surface analogies as the deepest level of truth, especially where words, expressions, or simple commonplace phenomena are discovered as evidence.

But if structural dichotomies are significant when contrasting occultic theorems with other ideologies, then the comparative personalities or psychologies of the creative individuals—the originators of these theorems—must be the most telling factors in separating the superstitiously eccentric "professor" from the professor who merely appears in his person or by his work to be uncommunicative, weird, or eccentric.

## *Weird versus Woebegone*

We have met Professor Rose. Now let us meet another pedagogue who superficially might appear just as bereft, both in action and philosophy. As a young man, *this* professor embarked on a habit of open-air exercises that included routinized peregrinations, rain or shine, at precisely half-past three every day, during which time he never spoke for fear of allowing infectious germs into his mouth. A philosopher at heart, he decided to apply his logical mind to the problem of keeping his stockings from sliding down his calves. He eventually accomplished this ideal by fastening his hose to elastic bands which he passed up under his trousers to his pockets, where they ended in springs contained in little boxes.

It took this person fifteen years to write his magnum opus; he finished it when he was fifty-seven years old. A startling book, it was full of long, intensive sentences alive with astonishing opinions about the mind, the universe, about something called a noumenon, and of what might be described in general as mental gymnastics par excellence.

For all intents and purposes, it seems that I have delineated another crackpot, who, though unsuperstitious by any test, seems as much taken with semantics and antics as any Edgar Cayce.

Of course, this is not the case at all, and the differentiation here between the ravings of Professor Rose and the towering genius of Immanuel Kant (the man with the springs in his pockets) is not only in the intellectual depth of one (Kant) and the sophistry of the other—those are but structural and textual diversities. The gap, above all, may be seen in the personality perspective. Rose is a frustrated, embittered, and distorted man who has turned to a militant form of superstitious harangue in order to assert himself, not as the inferior "loser" he unconsciously perceives himself to be, but as the world's true Messiah. Immanuel Kant, for all his eccentricities and probable neuroses, saw in his life's work a means of enlightening mankind, not aggrandizing himself. Whatever was "bugging him," to use the vernacular, it worked toward the production of original ideas, notable for their inspiration and pertinency. His philosophy, not his person, rose to prominence. The superstitious individual, however, cannot divorce his ego needs from his message and before long only the ego remains; the message is lost in a jumble that only the faithful—if any—can witness. Martin Luther, as another example, was saved from becoming simply a noisome eccentric by the intense and impersonal nature of his message. Though born of frustration, superstition, anger, and pride, the Lutheran doctrine neither sought to glorify Luther, per se, nor specifically to horrify the world (although it did horrify the Catholics). It was a saving principle offered as such. By contrast, Hitler's *Mein Kampf* teems with vindictive, self-glorifying allusions and details. Its purpose was clearly to function not as a light unto man, but as a universal demolition bomb.

The superstitious personality (and Hitler was surely one) is often driven by anger and eventually by revenge, which he hopes to translate in terms of power magically won. Surface eccentricities, turgid writings, and apparently revolutionary ideas are secondary to this violent frustration and should be studied only as symptomatic indications that may clarify related personality defects.

A schematic summary of the extreme cases we are discussing presents the following parallels. A strict religious upbringing generally leads to a reliance on biblical, religious, or other dogmatic quotations as the individual's exclusive expertise. Autistic or fantasy-ridden formularizations thereafter create a dependence on supernatural creatures and events as explanations of the world's design. At the same time, the individual's intellectual acuity, rejected by parents and friends because of its singularity, causes a process of awkward semantics, symbols, and freakish ideas to be applied to common evidence. Finally, the introverted repression that results from the characteristics so far described tends the young mind toward megalomaniacal attitudes of self-glorification (possibly leading to violence), all conceived in magical, power terms.

This summary represents, as noted, the extreme profile of the various types outlined in this book. In regard to the more positive and passive superstitious ideas presented at the beginning of this chapter, and in other chapters, the parallels take on minimalized qualities. In such cases, childhood is again dominated by religious pressure, but this is translated into a relatively poetic (though possibly gullible) expertise. Autism is precluded by simple daydreaming and self-propelling fantasy. The supernatural elements born of this tendency are fairly ephemeral and change as the perceiver matures; the goblins of childhood become the yahoos of urban life.

The minimally superstitious type is, by definition, less introverted, less repressed (if at all), and therefore disinclined to self-glorification or aggrandizement in its usual, overt forms. What, then, makes him superstitious at all, since he seems unrelated even slightly to the schema just presented? The answer lies in his intellect and idea formation, which inevitably lead to irrational applications and definitions, even in passive cases. This is the core of the superstitious character; the tendency to "read into," to decode, discover hidden (i.e., occultic) meanings, relationships, parallels, and departures; the "mental-gymnast" syndrome, which exerts itself on the bar bells of fantasy and myth in pursuit of easy magic. For whatever reason this type of mental procedure develops—and it may be due to early religious influence—it takes on this illogical (some might say poetic) "magicalism" causing WASHINGTON to mean "the cleansing of man by the year 2000," or any other similar concoction so far discussed. At best, such meanderings can satisfy certain psychic (that is nonphysical) needs, such as the reduction of nervous tension or the spurring of ambition and positive insight. But when faulty and degenerating, even in minimalized form, it can lead to outright sophism and gullibility, which in turn beckon exploitation and abuse.

## *Magicalism in Daily Life*

Each of us can appreciate the gymnastics of the full-blown superstitious type just rehearsed (mild *or* wild), since most of us also pursue, often indifferently, certain everyday attitudes and routines that fulfill a superstitious definition by assuming "easy magic" dimensions. In other words, we pursue these things in order to skip over the usual cause-and-effect requirements of a given situation. One will wear a lucky tie on a job interview in the secret hope that the tie will take care of the usually arduous and nerve-wracking aspects related to career.

I have separated four general categories of superstitious activity basic to almost every culture and individual. They do not clearly fall under the earlier rubrics and are, even when maximized, relatively harmless in terms of human psychology. Some of them, in fact, function as a crude but effective form of "positive thinking," particularly if employed by fairly well-adjusted individuals, those who know that it's "bad luck" to be superstitious.

### FLIRTATIONS WITH DESTINY

In these activities, the individual establishes a sort of *quid pro quo* with God (or the devil) or some superior force. "If I complete this business trip successfully, I'm going to clean out the cellar once and for all." What's implied, of course, is a hope that some higher power will graciously oversee and magically manipulate the various aspects of livelihood, in return for which, the happy businessman will feel obliged to undertake a particularly unpleasant, but tolerable, task (success on the job compensates and dignifies the cleanup). In most people's minds, prayer is a form of *quid pro quo* —and the more it tends toward "I'll do this, if you do that," the more superstitious is its formation.

### PICKING UP CLUES

This is a common form of omenizing in which we try to discover what may be (or what is) as a result of a particular simple happening. It's a sort of private game we play with ourselves to help us about a decision that has to be made or a problem resolved. "If the elevator door closes before I get to it, then it means I'm not going to have a pleasant weekend with the family." If the speaker wants to have a pleasant weekend, he may quicken his step in order to ensure an open elevator. If he needs a subconscious excuse for a quarrelsome family gathering (which he may have already programmed —or scripted), he will unwittingly slacken his pace. A common variant of this procedure is to egregiously relate cause and effect: "I lost out on this business opportunity today because I overate last night like a gluttonous pig." This attitude represents a sort of sin syndrome and takes on superstitious proportions in so far as one assumes that a kind of magical demerit book is being tallied on high.

## THE LITTLE RITUALS

Among the most intensive, unconscious activities most of us pursue are those little routines or rituals that we presume, often without knowing it, will magically aid in some endeavor. It is this *magic* factor, of course, which defines the superstitious inclination of most such routines. Benjamin Franklin conceived an elaborate ritual for getting to bed (and thus to sleep—a process that often requires some form of "magic"). "When . . . you find you cannot sleep easily . . ." he wrote, "get out of bed, beat up and turn your pillow, shake the bed clothes well at least twenty shakes, then throw the bed open and leave it to cool . . ."[5]

My own prebed ritual includes (frequently) a quick listen at the household intercom, which picks up street noises at the main door. The crackling static seems to have a soothing effect. But, in fact, it simply reassures me that all is well with the world and therefore I may be allowed to rest. Franklin's procedure was similarly useful since a neat, cool bed is all the more conducive to comfort and eventually sleep.

Other daily rituals include systems of dressing, checking for locked doors and windows, placing the change in one pocket as opposed to the other, eating certain foods in a certain way (vegetables consumed separately from meat), and so forth down the line. When extremely compulsive, of course, these idiosyncracies can lead to neurotic problems; not all are superstitious either, but some become so deeply rooted and so necessary to a particular function that they evolve into personalized forms of "knocking on wood."

IT CREEPS UP ON YOU

There are simple habits which begin to be associated with specific events and actions and therefore seem indispensable for carrying through an act. In a way such things relate to the trinkets fondly worn by Trinketeers (Chapter 3). For example, a writer I knew used to squeeze a soft rubber eraser in his left hand while writing with his right. He had developed this tension-reducing habit in lieu of smoking. As such it was a good thing. Superstitious considerations developed when he began to assume that he couldn't write without the eraser stuck between the fingers of his left hand. Somehow that lump of gray latex had become his muse and he nervously secured it in place (like a talisman) before each bout with paper and pencil.

A charming, and true, story in this vein demonstrates a form of tradition building, which perfectly applies as well to the development of superstitions. One of the greatest operatic tenors of the nineteenth century was Francesco Tamagno, who created the title role in Verdi's *Otello*. So masterful was Tamagno's interpretation of this part that it became a standard for tenors throughout the world. One day, a few years after *Otello*'s première, a younger tenor came to Tamagno to pay homage and revealed how he faithfully imitated every single detail of the master's performance. "There is however," he said, "one gesture that confuses me as to motivation, even though I do it faithfully."

"What is that?" asked Tamagno.

"It occurs in the second act," the young man answered, "just before the big 'Now and Forever Farewell' aria. You go to the rear of the stage, your back to the audience, you jerk your head forward, and seem to be surveying the scenery for no obvious reason at all."

The great tenor seemed perplexed, thought for a moment, then finally exclaimed: "Oh yes, of course! That's when I go back there in order to spit."

Tamagno's expectoration had become a cherished operatic tradition very much like wearing a rabbit's foot or covering mirrors after funerals or a thousand other such superstitious things. We do them faithfully, though few know why. And when we do find out, it all boils down to some simple, if not simplistic, and very human explanation—such as Signor Tamagno's clearing his phlegm.

CHAPTER 9

# *Toward a Psychology of Superstition*

Generally speaking, clinical correlation of superstitious beliefs and neurotic behavior is not a frequent practice among psychotherapists or other counselors of the disturbed. This is surprising considering the detailed biography most analysts attempt to develop with patients or potential patients. By and large, these biographies may include only passing references to the subject's belief patterns, although they stress rather heavily, and no doubt correctly, other influential conscious or subconscious ideas: sex, career security, and family interrelationships being significant among them. In other words, integrated religious experiences as part of the over-all personality interview have not been developed, even though advocated by William James as early as 1902.

This is not to imply that the subject at hand has not concerned psychologists over the years. Freud wrote about superstition, or what he called "faulty actions," and Carl Jung is said to have drawn horoscopes of his patients, apparently in deference to their own beliefs. But Freud's concern in this area was in analyzing unconscious formulations—why the mind inclined thus and so as a result of certain stimuli. And much evidence suggests that Jung did not chart the astrological profile of his patients because he wanted to know what *they* believed, but because he himself believed that astrology was a valid part of his elaborate notion of synchronicity—or multiple influences coinciding at a given time. Jung, in fact, became, as a result of his intensive studies of occultic archetypes, something of a "haunted man." He is said to have asserted, among other things, that Freud's physical presence in his study caused various books to psychokinetically leap or fly from their bookcase shelves.

Neither Freud nor Jung nor William James nor many contemporary therapists and researchers in psychology specifically evaluate superstitious beliefs (or any beliefs) as symptomatic evidence in tandem with psychoneurosis. In other words, they do not study what I have called credology (or systematic belief patterns) in the profile of the individual with anything near the concern they manifest, for example, over dream interpretation or early sexual conduct. No one is deprecating either the meaning of dreams or sex in the profile of a patient; these investigations are as essential in mental therapy as are blood pressure or metabolism tests in physical medicine. But I think it can eventually be shown that an individual's deeply inculcated horror of Satan, as one example, or belief in astral projection or dependence on trinkets for coping with life are equally pertinent to psychoanalysis and general mental-health therapy.

Two relatively historical failings are responsible for an apparent prejudice among psychologists concerning the elements of credology as symptomologic evidence. In the first place, psychologists and physicians have almost no training whatsoever in such subjects as comparative religion, theology, mythology, or cultural anthropology, in which details of superstitious or occult beliefs are usually discussed. One can hardly blame them for this lapse in curriculum emphasis; it is a problem of programming in colleges and universities. Besides, except for strictly objective courses in comparative religion (which is a fairly new field), and the even rarer objective study of the occult, most schools do not really provide interdisciplinary studies in human belief patterns, whether specifically religious, folkloric, or metaphysical in content. Would-be psychologists simply cannot, in the regular course of their studies, learn precisely what a Catholic believes, or why a superstitious person fears broken mirrors, or the socio-psychological tangents of ritual, theism, eschatology, and any other dimension of credology.

On top of this, there prevails in the West, and especially in America, a sort of taboo about discussing other people's beliefs, particularly religious, because they are usually considered sacrosanct and "none of your business." A sort of First Amendment inversion applies to any evaluation that may touch on religious background or worship or even on someone's atheistic philosophies. This general attitude is probably born out of a justified concern that discriminatory consequences may follow such knowledge. It would be unfortunate indeed if we "punished" a political candidate, or anyone else, for that matter, for his religious affiliations, particularly if they are casual or superficial, as many are these days. But a potential president who is deeply involved with horoscopes or is a devout Mormon, for example, supports beliefs that will clearly color his life, possibly in a positive way, possibly not, and they should not be ignored or swept under a carpet of propriety.

Even so, of the three "personal" subjects once forbidden in discussion at every bar or cocktail party—sex, politics, and religion—only religion, that is, belief, remains relatively untouchable, even to analysts, possibly because of persuasive First Amendment ideas. Such inhibitions notwithstanding, it should be evident that as surely as a political figure's intense opinions on God and the devil (or the stars) may be useful items to know in forming an intelligent evaluation of his fitness for office, then how much more valuable and essential should be such considerations as regards the psychoneurotic patient or potential patient. In fact, in evaluating our own personalities and in pursuing the modern discipline of "finding out who I am," these credological concerns must be likewise viewed with urgency and relevance. By ignoring, for whatever reason, the role of belief, or nonbelief, in personality and behavior, we are overlooking a fundamental ingredient in the human and social mix.

## Credology Clues

A therapist with whom I was speaking after a lecture I gave on the deeper meaning of the recent *Exorcist* reaction told me that one of his patients, a young man about twenty-three, "was acting out the heavy fantasy that he was a witch." I asked the doctor what he thought this meant in the over-all terms of the patient's problem, which he had not yet articulated to me. "It's just a fantasy," the therapist replied, "probably related to antisocial reactions that he employs as defensive mechanisms."

"How did the subject of witchcraft first come up?" I asked. The therapist thought for a moment. "Oh yes, we were discussing his weekly routine and he mentioned that he attended witch Sabbats on occasion, 'all except on Tuesdays,' that is. He seemed most insistent on avoiding Tuesday Sabbats."

Taking on a bit of a Sherlock Holmes air, I asked: "Do you suspect that this patient is troubled by repressed homoerotic conflicts?" The doctor's eyes widened and he nodded energetically. "Why yes; many things point in that direction. But how did you know?"

"In the fantasies of modern witches," I told him, "there is a notion that Tuesday Sabbats, for some obscure reason, are devoted to sodomy, fellatio, and homosexual rites. Anyone who believed in witchcraft, but who struggled to repress homosexual expression would probably assiduously avoid those rituals."

The doctor was impressed with this unusual and significant bit of evidence. Had he known this sort of thing from a credological study of witchcraft, he might have been able to corroborate his prognosis earlier and thus, by now, have begun effective treatment for his patient.

In some cases, intelligent application of belief patterns to outward behavior are revealed by common sense. Arthur Lyons (in *The Second Coming: Satanism in America*), who as far as I know is not a psychotherapist, relates the fantasy of astral projection to the ego perception of a young, unattractive male Satanist "of runtish build," with "a nice collection of pimples . . . [whose] jaunts into astral projection were . . . an escape from a physical realm he found to be a burden rather than a pleasure."[1] This perceptive analysis relates quite nicely to the Dualist's (or Satanist's) either/or mentality (corporeal body versus astral body) and the Seer's inability or unwillingness to accept obvious and tangible explanations for obstensibly "out-of-body, out-of-mind" experiences.

With functional integration of the information set forth in this book, the therapist or the individual himself can now proceed to study what might be called basic superstitious signals, and thus rate patients (or himself) according to the types and intensities earlier outlined. What follows is a sort of do-it-yourself procedure for just this kind of analysis in terms of superstitions as they might possibly relate to mental health, both positively and negatively. Such a scheme is only meant to be indicative and if the individual feels that greater problems are manifested by the tendencies he discovers, consultation with professional psychologists or counselors should be immediately undertaken.

## *Which Type Are You?*

1. If you tend to propitiate by sacrificial acts supposedly negative supernatural forces, you may be what I have called an *Appeaser*. The minimal example given for this type is the common habit of knocking on wood to demonstrate respect for ancient pagan tree-gods; it is an action usually performed without much conscious thought. When accompanied by casual lighthearted sentiments, it passes for a social ritual that indicates recognition of enigmatic forces in nature (the ups and downs of life), and if you do it for positive reasons, it should provide you with unconscious satisfaction and a sense of deference that frequently helps to bolster productive attitudes. Your motivation at such times may be the following idea: "I respect the vagaries of life and am not truly as arrogant and unfeeling as I seem. Therefore I may hope that good fortune will smile upon me."

However, when compulsiveness characterizes this particular appeasing attitude, when you feel obliged to pay craven obeisance to fate, you may actually be signaling a frightened tendency toward unconscious and destructive self-sacrifice. This tendency is usually based on a childhood fear of "losing out" because of some hidden, threatening force in nature. In extreme cases, sacrifice of simple physical function (like psychologically induced paralysis), of family or social serenity, or of some tangible asset or possession (cracking up a new car, for instance) may follow in a desperate though unconscious attempt to forestall the menacings of fate, nature, or even of the gods.

Was fear of nature inculcated in you during childhood? Were you told: "Thunder means that God is angry with you . . ." and thoughts like that? If so, you must come to recognize anew the fact that primitive and man-made fallacies have invested nature with humanlike attributes and temperament (wrath, vengeance, and so forth) that have no place in reality or common sense. Only by deflating the "unknown" forces that you assume require propitiation and humility can you help reduce the appeasing compulsion and its resultant sacrificial demands.

2. Is your view of life dominated by a conflict in which, perennially, good versus evil (God versus Satan) and which often de-

mands that you choose sides at some critical point in life? If so, you may be a *Dualist*, in which case you were probably raised in a strict religious way (no matter what you may have later become). The operative question that defines the scope of your Dualist attitude is this (and you may ask it of yourself): "Do I believe that there are extraneous forces outside my own responsibility that govern all my good and evil actions? Further, do I regard the cosmos as either purely hostile or purely benevolent?"

Minimally effected, the Dualist disposition—which affirmatively answers the questions just asked—tends to rely on the hope that God, or good, will be eventually triumphant over ostensible evil. If you feel this way, then you probably believe that demons are a sort of symbolic reality; a sort of religious (as opposed to scientific) fact. Unfortunately, such a belief, though comparatively moderate, tends to cement you to certain early religious fantasies that may conflict with your intellectual desire to acknowledge a more rational, "grown-up" view. The conflict of these beliefs naturally enhances the endemic dualism of this neurosis. Consequently, you may find yourself more and more tolerant of belief in demon possession and, at the same time, you may begin to perceive a viable view of Satan and his hordes. Eventually, you might even come to prefer the "company" of fiends to the usual speculations about God. Specific advocacy of Satanism is the logical terminus of this type of thinking.

In general, Dualist superstitions are usually maximized and rarely passive, leading to "possession" manias, as well as schizoid reactions; the so-called "Jekyll-Hyde" syndrome. When extreme, this behavior can destroy the usual values of right and wrong and thus encourage antisocial or criminal activities. Homicidal psychosis, severe anguish, and fantasies regarding the devil, or the devil versus God, are often revealed in reports from the police.

By demythologizing in your own mind the entire Satan story and preventing its wild-eyed inculcation among the young, you will be able to diminish this explosive and very current aberration. A hint: how you reacted to the film version of *The Exorcist* or to other similar realizations of Satan and his works may be a sort of litmus-paper test for judging your superstitious aptitude vis-à-vis dualism and its snares.

3. Do you seek tangible symbolic forms that you believe can bring you, by contact, either luck or love, health or financial power?

Do you wear jewelry as some sort of talisman? Are you fond of amulets, believing them to possess "natural vibes" of magic? What of clothing, perfumes, or other objects (a car, a favorite chair)? Do they contain, in your opinion, luck-giving or magical powers? If you can answer yes to these questions, no doubt you incline toward the superstitions of the *Trinketeer*. When minimal and therefore least neurotic, your fancies may be taken simply as a cultural phenomenon. A tendency to dependence, however, to the transference of responsibility to the particular trinket or charm and a development of intensely materialistic interpersonal attitudes born of fixation on "things," bodes trouble and may lead you to a crass object-evaluation of persons, philosophies, and life itself. In such circumstances, you may catch yourself saying, "Unless someone has blue eyes, perfect teeth, and radiant health, I'm not going to get involved and spoil my own luck any more than I would purposely leave behind my lucky beads or 'magic' scarf . . ."

As counteraction in this area, which can be quite costly as well as ridiculous, you should try to de-emphasize superstition in general, meaning supernaturalism, magic, and the occult. By doing so, you will enable a cross, for example, to be what it was supposed to be—a symbol of a particular belief and not a protective device invested with magic. Any protective magic has got to be within you, not residing in a hunk of metal or a dried-out rabbit's foot. For the heck of it, try leaving your "lucky" charm at home one day when you venture out into the world. Then be objective; see if your "luck" really has been affected and try to gauge just how much of your own subconscious scripting is responsible for your everyday scenarios.

4. A problem with sexual insecurity or an inadequate sense of self may drive you to certain medieval delusions born of sorcery and withcraft, both of which seem to promise power and glamor. If you find yourself addicted to the hocus-pocus of such beliefs, you probably fall into the *Conjuror* category. It may be, of course, a passing addiction or fascination with the antics of witchery. You may even welcome an occasional fling at coven sex, in which oddball rituals are employed as a "turn on." Is this your "thing"? So be it—these are hardly indicative of psychoneurosis, although they may bespeak a rather groveling level of taste.

When the abracadabra of ersatz withcraft becomes indispensable for your arousal, or when artificial notions about your own magical prowess and allurement dominate libidinous desires, then your superstition has become fixed and troublesome. You are in danger of depersonalization, habitual eccentricity, and exploitation; in short, the Conjuror's confusion.

Women Conjurors may be so confused in this vein that once they are inducted into the secrets of sorcery they find themselves falling back on promiscuity as a "proof" of power. Men under the same enthrallment may tend to be abusive or compulsively drawn to impersonal sex and possibly sado-masochistic rituals. If this type of thing is already your *modus operandi,* beware. The "kinky" soon replaces sincere and dependable sex stimuli, deepening the habit of ritualized eroticism. This habit can eventually lead to failure of performance as you begin to see yourself realistically in the preposterous posture of an erotic clown.

Those fascinated by Conjuror bewitchment or grandiose promises of power open themselves to easy seduction and abuse, particularly because their motivations in the first place are founded on insecurity in sexual areas. To test this tendency, you should ask yourself if you easily accept, even in principle, the magical formulas and claims proffered by so-called witches. Can you distinguish between basic exhibitionistic erotic behavior and what are supposed to be "supernatural" powers of love? Do you like to ritualize sex or sexual fantasies and see yourself as a power figure, priest or priestess of "amor"?

You may say no to each of the above and yet be Conjuror material, especially if you must rely on love magic and ritual even passively (becoming a "slave" of the priest or priestess mentioned above). Should this occur, you might come to feel responsible only to the laws of witchcraft and sorcery as opposed to your inner feelings and sense of propriety. This, in the long run, is simply a form of self-delusion, which casts you in the role of what might be called a witchcraft "groupie."

A whole spectrum of psychosexual difficulties surrounds Conjuror superstitions and presses dangerously close to Dualist concerns for Satanism and antisocial behavior. Again, depropagandizing the mythical powers of witches and their conjurations is essential for you in reversing the type of aberrant activity which confuses ritual with power and eroticism with love.

5. Almost everyone experiences a certain neurotic displacement

when confronted with the loss of a loved one, and morbid tendencies are not unusual at certain ages or in the context of crisis and fear. A plethora of funerary rituals and gestures serves well in the early hours of loss to help diminish the shock and sense of tragedy by conversely stimulating expressions of grief. But there are those— you may be among them—who, burdened by unreasonable guilt and seeking recrimination, begin to cower beneath spectral threats and accusations until the world is "peopled" by ghosts and ghostly superstitions. Such is the *Expiator's* world. It is not just the realm of bereavement. Those who prefer to wear a black armband or black stockings for thirty days (or even sixty days) as a demonstration of their loss and/or grief probably reinforce eventual adjustment by this symbolic act. But if you, like Queen Victoria, prefer to be holed up in your "widow's weeds" for over a decade, this clearly exemplifies aberrant superstitious behavior.

Compulsion born of irrational guilt concerning the deceased is the basis of psychoneurotic reaction in the Expiator's category. Some symptoms of this problem are revealed by a broad range of superstitions relating to the return of the dead and the reality of spirits, ghosts, emanations, and the like. If, as a result of your loss, you believe in such things, you might also find yourself "conversing" with the dear departed, promising penance and a form of living death in exchange for expiation.

All such confrontations involving loss and death that summon up fantasies of ghosts, reincarnation, spectral visitations, and related bugaboos are indicative of a deeply troubled attitude that may drive the Expiator into a living tomb of paranoidal withdrawal and terror. If this is your tendency, you should avoid, like the plague, the current emphasis on hauntings, spiritualism, and the implications of reincarnation and simplistic, untheological nonsense about the afterlife and the destiny of man's soul. These ideas only tend to stimulate Expiator anxieties and the renunciation of a meaningful life that often follows such anxieties.

6. If you are what I call a *Stargazer*, you probably feel a need to fantasize scientifically in order to regimentate an otherwise shaky life. As a result, astrology greatly appeals to you, although all forms of cosmic superstition involving the supernatural or the mysterious fall under similar stargazing propensities. Do you, for example, find yourself more and more dependent on the promise of extra-

terrestrial saviors, or the reappearance of Atlantis, or the effects of the moon on your specific emotions? Or is it a compulsive interest in horoscopes, sun signs, UFOs, and the like that captivates your fancy? You might have cause to worry about such things unless you can honestly say that they help stimulate further study in valid, scientific areas such as astronomy or space technology thus providing a minimal form of discipline in what you think to be a chaotic life.

When carried to extremes, these ideas develop into a compulsive religiosity concerning astrology and its related conceits. You can see this coming by testing the discipline you seek in this area to see if it soon turns to restraint and inhibition, including manic-type moods unconsciously based on your changing "chart" or horoscope (up one day, down the next). Or have you ever experienced quasi-paranoid relationships with family and friends, owing to what you consider their "favorable aspects" or "unfavorable trines"? Do situations arise in which your career might be jeopardized by unconscious desires to fail which are expressed in pessimistic readings of astrological cant? Have you, in short, become a stargazing slave? If your answer to any of these questions is yes, you may find that eventually such thinking leads to mental rigidity and fatalism, reinstating your worst infantile fears about drifting off in space and all the other alienations that first turned your eyes to the stars in such dependent myopia.

You'll probably agree that debunking the scientific allegations of astrology and other space superstitions will do precious little to offset their influences on you. Should this be the case, you require more subtle transference to less undependable and confusing forms of discipline like athletics or a health-club regimen. Under such sensible routines, you may be able to forestall complete surrender to the jumble of words, symbols, and conceits that make up the usual practices of Stargazers.

7. Do you see yourself as a master of time and space and all uncertainty? Can you omenize or read anything into everything? At the same time, do you find there is a block in you when it comes to looking inward to your own unconscious motivations for what appear to be psychic powers? Those who answer positively to these questions must consider themselves denizens of the category peopled by *Seers*. It is perhaps the most highly developed category

of superstitious types, replete as it is with often amazing feats of self-deception and nearly artistic manipulations and embellishments of coincidence, natural talent (including legerdemain), and normal perceptivity.

If you are a Seer, you operate within the general field of the psychic, but only as it concerns the supernatural or otherworldly dimensions. You do not "dig" the statistical and comparatively insipid programs of parapsychology and experimentation, except as "proof" of your beliefs. These beliefs include "seeing" into the future, reading palms, numbers, tea leaves, or cards and performing a wide repertoire of apparently superphenomenal or psychic acts (generally labeled *psi,* or inexplicable).

Yours may be minimal Seer-like inclinations or flirtations with unrecognized talents of deduction and insight. Do you invariably assume such talents to be forms of "extrasensory perception"? Or can you ever bring yourself to admit that the "extra" factor in such ESP experiences does not necessarily imply supernaturalism? If you can, you may avoid a plunge into the superstitious pitfalls of the Seer delusion. Those who fail to avoid these traps, those who come to rely on prophecy and Tarot cards as opposed to self-confidence and native skills, may fall prey to professionals in the field who, these days, have attained nearly godlike staus. Perhaps you are attracted to such types—the mind readers, key benders, and feedback "freaks." Unfortunately, your fascination is fraught with danger, since you may end up being exploited by these people in everything from your view of personal liberty to your physical health. In the last category, a series of destructive mental delusions can develop when you begin to replace personal responsibility for your actions with the blandishments of psychicism. These problems include out-of-body fantasies, psychedelic hallucination, drug use, and bouts of acute egomania.

The individual who unflinchingly accepts the antinatural premises of precognition, psychokinesis, and the like may well be on the way to total delusion. Dr. Albert Ellis states that ". . . one of the requisites for emotional health is acceptance of uncertainty . . ."2 Unless you can accept this axiom, even in principle, you may be a candidate for the Seer neurosis. Hint: deflating the superstars of this realm—the pop-culture Seers—can go a long way toward reversing the irrational confusion that they provoke among those who are hung upon uncertainties.

## *Clinic versus Coven*

There should be no shame or sense of belittlement felt by those who may fall into the extreme, or even moderate, definitions of the types just summarized. Superstitious neurosis like any other form of maladjustment should bear no opprobrium in sensible, compassionate minds. Developing from trauma, from certain forms of abuse and faulty education, for which the individual cannot be blamed, this type of maladjustment, more than most, is reinforced by the pressures and stresses of daily life which tend to unsettle practically everyone at some point or another. After all, the inability properly to reconcile stress with inherent psychological weaknesses is a universal fact and can be compared to the problems of sleeplessness caused by the noise of low-flying airplanes. If we cannot sleep, our systems weaken; as a result we may soon fall prey to viruses and other health disorders. Just as there is absolutely nothing reprehensible about catching the flu, so there must be no secrecy or shame about even the most medieval anxieties or maladjustments. At the same time, not taking care of the illness or trouble when it becomes obvious, or "spreading" it around, so to speak, is, of course, untenable and self-destructive, as well as potentially antisocial.

A recent case, so glaring and so unbelieveable that it appears to be a Hollywood creation, reveals the extremes to which superstitious psychoneurosis can go. It is reported here and not in the Dualist chapter, where it also belongs, because of its public concern with the psychiatric aspects of what we have been discussing throughout this book. The report comes out of England, where I fear a new wave of superstitionism, particularly of the Dualist-Conjuror sort, threatens to become a second Bubonic plague.

Near Barnsley, in the English Midlands, in October 1974, a certain Michael Taylor brutally tore his wife to pieces, tore out her eyes and her tongue, and according to testimony at his trial in Leeds, "tore her face almost off and she died very quickly from inhalation of blood." The murderer's motivation was possession. Both he and his wife, he believed, had been overwhelmed by Satan. Believing this, they had earlier thrown themselves on the mercy of local exorcists, including two clergymen, who proceeded to purge the thirty-one-year-old Taylor of over "forty evil spirits" residing in his soul. Unfortunately, as Taylor himself confessed, the exorcists "had tried to bring me peace of mind. But instead, they filled me with the devil. I was [therefore] compelled by the forces within me to destroy everything in our house."

So it was that one morning Taylor found himself stalking naked through the streets near his home, covered in what he called "Satan's blood," but which was, in fact, the blood of his mutilated wife.

The prosecutor at the trial lamented, "It is perhaps astonishing in this day and age [that] they [the exorcists] all came to the conclusion that Taylor was possessed by Satan, by a strong force of evil which required nothing more or less than prolonged exorcism." What the murderer really required, another speaker said, was "to be in a psychiatric unit."[3] But this suggestion was rejected by the exorcists when they first examined Taylor's case because they felt it was more in line with the sufferer's superstitious disease to proceed to superstitious cures and the casting out of forty devils.

The court at Leeds ruled otherwise and in March 1975 declared Taylor insane and committed him, finally, to a mental hospital.


## A Sound Mind

Any symptoms that signal disorder of our health and equilibrium, our mental adjustment or general abilities, must be taken seriously whether the symptoms are suspicious lumps or irrational dependence on the supernatural excesses of superstitious belief. It may possibly sound alarmist to warn against the dangers of certain superstitious beliefs and tendencies as though they were in fact elements of disease. But this I have done, and I believe it must be done against the background of contemporary culture, which more and more begins to resemble, in the words of Theodore Roszak, a "cultic hothouse . . . where every manner of mystery and fakery, ritual and rite, intermingle with marvelous indiscrimination."[4]

Who or what is at fault in this mishmash of credology is the subject of another book. This effort, however, has been undertaken to delineate and scrutinize the broad scope of superstition as it relates to human conduct and psychology. I believe one may conclude that this scrutiny has revealed, with notable positive exceptions, that superstitious, that is, irrational and occultic, dependencies are inimical to the sensible life and may be symptomatic of psychoneurotic illness in varying degrees. An attempt to relate these superstitions to specific sources in history and thereby to demythologize their putative supernatural origins has also been pursued in these pages in the belief that awareness of the limitations and of the human dimensions of what was formerly thought to be extraordinary magic will go a long way to diminishing the glamor and seductiveness of superstitious conceits.

The true magic in our lives is the radiant combination of reasonableness and sensitivity that produces both civilization and the chance for expressive personal freedom. In turn, that freedom enlivens our own individual responsibilities, our autonomy, integrity, our self-respect, potentials, and native talents. Conversely, false dependence on fictional beliefs, on cults, fads, and the like, with their facile promises of quick power, easy solution, and fleeting gratification, in the long run leads only to a form of slavery. To put it more poetically, perhaps, the flight from reason is invariably a flight from freedom.

And so it is worth repeating: knocking on wood may be a casual, even lighthearted deference to a higher force—a force which each of us must eventually contemplate. But essentially, for the truest benefit of all, we should knock within, on the doors of our conscious and unconscious treasuries. At the same time, we must constantly work to purge irrational anxiety either by dint of our own efforts or with professional guidance and help. The goal is tranquillity, strength, and optimism. It is for many a very realistic goal, for as one may read in II Timothy 1:7, "God hath not given us the Spirit of fear; but of power, and of love, and of a sound mind."

# Notes

## Introduction

1. Francis Bacon: *Of Superstition,* quoted in *Dictionary of Quotations,* ed. B. Evans, p. 671.
2. Edmund Burke: "Reflections on the Revolution in France," quoted in ibid., p. 671.
3. Sigmund Freud: *The Basic Writings of,* p. 165.
4. Thomas Hobbes: *Leviathan I,* quoted in *Dictionary of Quotations,* p. 580.
5. *Encyclopedia Britannica,* 1962, Vol. 21, p. 557(b).
6. Trevor Ravenscroft: *The Spear of Destiny,* Bantam Books, New York, N.Y., 1974, p. xiv.

## Chapter 1

1. Sigmund Freud: *The Basic Writings of,* p. 150.
2. James Frazer: *The Golden Bough* (Macmillan ed.), p. 805.
3. Anita Mühl: "Automatic Writing . . ." in *Outline of Abnormal Psychology,* ed. G. Murphy, p. 213.
4. Alfred Adler: *Understanding Human Nature,* p. 235.

## Chapter 2

1. Anton S. La Vey: *The Satanic Bible,* pp. 52–53.
2. Ambassador College Publication: *The Occult Explosion,* 1973–74, p. 35, p. 40.
3. Ibid., p. 40.

4. C. S. Lewis: *The Screwtape Letters* (Macmillan paperback), p. vii.
5. Ibid., p. 172.
6. Charles Francis Potter: *The Story of Religion*, Garden City Publishing Co., Inc., Garden City, N.Y., 1929, p. 80.
7. Ibid, p. 80.
8. Clyde Z. Nunn: quoted in *Time* magazine, April 29, 1974, p. 99.
9. Billy Graham: quoted in *The National Enquirer*, summer 1974.
10. Pope Paul VI: quoted in New York *Times*, December 18, 1972, p. 16.
11. Ibid.
12. Eugene Kennedy: quoted in New York *Times*, January 28, 1974, p. 15.
13. Andrew M. Greeley: quoted in New York *Times Magazine*, February 4, 1973, p. 12.
14. Samuel De Nicola: quoted in New York *Daily News*, March 16, 1974, p. 4.
15. Robert L. Stevenson: *The Strange Case of Dr. Jekyll and Mr. Hyde* (Dodd, Mead), p. 53.
16. Advertisement in *The Village Voice*, April 18, 1974, p. 19.
17. Ibid.
18. Herbert A. Aikins: "Casting out a Stuttering Devil," in *The Outline of Abnormal Psychology*, ed. Gardner Murphy, the Modern Library, Inc., New York, N.Y. 1929, p. 175.
19. News story in Toronto *Star*, February 24, 1975, p. 1, p. A4.
20. Richard T. Janssen: News story in *Wall Street Journal*, December 10, 1974, p. 1.
21. News story in *Sunday Telegraph* (London), quoted in ibid.
22. Janssen, loc. cit.
23. Albert Schweitzer: *The Quest for the Historical Jesus*, Macmillan Co., New York, N.Y., 1968, p. 398.

## Chapter 3

1. Emile de Givry: *Witchcraft, Magic and Alchemy*, University Books, New Hyde Park, N.Y., 1958, p. 340.
2. Carl Gustav Jung: *Man and His Symbols*, p. 243.
3. James Frazer: *The Golden Bough*, p. 405.
4. William Inge: *Come Back Little Sheba*, Random House, Inc., New York, N.Y., 1949.

## Chapter 4


1. Ed Sanders: "Charlie and the Devil," in *Esquire* magazine, November 1973, p. 235.
2. Louise Huebner: *Power Through Witchcraft*, Bantam Books, New York, N.Y., 1971, flyleaf.
3. Private correspondence in author's files. January 1972.
4. Margaret A. Murray: *The Witch-Cult in Western Europe*, p. 279.
5. Jules Michelet: *Satanism and Witchcraft*, p. 87.
6. Ibid., p. 88.
7. Pennethorne Hughes: *Witchcraft*, p. 87.
8. Colin Wilson: *The Occult*, p. 51.
9. ———: in New York *Times*, November 6, 1971, Op-ed page.
10. Arthur Lyons: *The Second Coming: Satanism in America*, p. 128.
11. Gérard Bonnot: "La Sorcière du C.n.r.s" in *L'Express* magazine, p. 57.
12. Edward J. Moody: "Magical Therapy: Contemporary Satanism," in *Religious Movements in Contemporary America*, ed I. I. Zaretsky and M. P. Leone, p. 359.


## Chapter 5


1. Ross Thalheimer: *Reflections*, p. 151.
2. Gaston Maspero: *Ancient Egypt and Assyria*, D. Appleton and Co., New York, N.Y. 1910, p. 118.
3. Maxim Gorky: *Enemies:* a Play, trans. Jeremy Brooks and Kitty Hunter-Blair, Viking Press, 1972.
4. A. D. Coleman: "Spirit Photographs: Are They Hoaxes?" in New York *Times*, June 4, 1972.
5. Arthur Ford (as told to James Ellison): "The Life Beyond Death," reprinted in New York *Daily News*, January 19, 1972, p. 44.
6. James Frazer: *The Golden Bough*, p. 401.


## Chapter 6


1. Arthur Koestler: quoted in New York *Times*, July 21, 1969, p. 21.
2. Pablo Picasso: quoted in ibid., p. 21.
3. Gloria Doyle: verbatim on CBS-TV, Syracuse, N.Y., March 12, 1975.

4. Carl Gustav Jung: quoted in *Encyclopedia of Magic and Superstition*, ed. Richard Cavendish, p. 66.
5. Linda Goodman: *Sun Signs*, Bantam Books, Inc., New York, N.Y., 1971, p. 123.
6. Helen Gurley Brown, ed: *Cosmopolitan Guide to Fortunetelling*, 1974, p. 162.
7. Christopher Lyon and James Stephenson: "An Astrological Study of Coronary Heart Disease," in *The Aquarian Agent*, August 1970, p. 16.
8. Erich Fromm: *Escape from Freedom*, p. 217.
9. Carl Sagan: "Unidentified Flying Object" in *Encyclopedia Americana*, 1970, Vol. 27, p. 369.
10. Private correspondence in author's files, 1973.
11. Mary Ellen Carter: *Edgar Cayce on Prophecy*, p. 52.


## *Chapter 7*


1. Aleister Crowley: *The Confessions of*, p. 110.
2. Isaac Bashevis Singer: quoted in New York *Times Magazine*, March 25, 1975.
3. Sigmund Freud: quoted in *Psychology and Extrasensory Perception*, ed. Raymond Van Over, p. 111.
4. Mary Ellen Carter: *Edgar Cayce on Prophecy*, p. 93.
5. Jeane Dixon: quoted in *National Star*, August 3, 1974, p. 11.
6. Ibid.
7. Norman Rush: "You Gotta Believe!" in *The Village Voice*, September 12, 1974, p. 22.
8. Ibid., p. 24.
9. Jacob Bronowski: verbatim on "The Ascent of Man," television series, PBS Network, 1975.
10. Eileen J. Garrett: *Sense and Nonsense of Prophecy*, p. 13.
11. Private correspondence in author's files, 1973.
12. Francis Bacon: *Novum Organum (I)*, quoted in *Dictionary of Quotations*, ed. B. Evans, p. 452.


## *Chapter 8*


1. Private correspondence in author's files, 1974.
2. Morton Prince: in *An Outline of Abnormal Psychology*, p. 532.
3. Isaac Asimov: "The Planet That Wasn't," in *Fantasy and Science Fiction Magazine*, May 1975, p. 109.

4. "Professor Rose": uncopyrighted material, 1973.
5. Benjamin Franklin: quoted in *Insomnia* by Gay Gaer Luce and Dr. Julius Segal, Doubleday & Co., Inc., Garden City, N.Y., 1969, p. 182.

## Chapter 9

1. Arthur Lyons: *The Second Coming: Satanism in America*, p. 156.
2. Albert Ellis: *The Case Against Religion: A Psychotherapist's View*, Institute for Rational Living, New York, N.Y., 1965, p. 16.
3. Harry Trimborn: "A Simple Man Turns Killer," in New York *Post*, March 15, 1975, p. 20.
4. Theodore Roszak: quoted in *The Humanist* magazine, September–October 1974, p. 25.

# Recommended Reading


ADLER, ALFRED. *Understanding Human Nature*. Garden City, N.Y.: Star Books, 1927.

ALLPORT, GORDON W. *Personality*. New York: Henry Holt & Co., 1937.

ASIMOV, ISAAC. *Asimov's Mysteries*. New York: Doubleday & Co., 1968.

BONNOT, GÉRARD. "La Sorcière du C.n.r.s." *L'Express*, Paris, August 19–25, 1974.

BRASCH, R. *How Did It Begin?* New York: David McKay, 1966.

BREASTED, JAMES. *The Dawn of Conscience*. New York: Charles Scribner's Sons, 1935.

BROWN, NORMAN O. *Life Against Death*. New York: Vintage Books, 1959.

BURLAND, C. A. *Myths of Life and Death*. New York: Crown Publishers, 1974.

CAMPBELL, JOSEPH. *The Masks of God: Primitive Mythology*. New York: Viking Press, 1962.

CARTER, MARY ELLEN. *Edgar Cayce on Prophecy*. New York: Paperback Library, Inc., 1968.

CASARIL, GUY. *La Magie Quotidienne*. Paris: Société des Editions Modernes, 1962.

CASTANEDA, CARLOS. *The Teachings of Don Juan*. Los Angeles: Univ. of California Press, 1968.

CAVENDISH, RICHARD. *The Black Arts*. New York: Capricorn Books, 1968.

———, ed. *Man, Myth and Magic*. New York: Marshall Cavendish Corp., 1970.

CIRLOT, J. E. *Dictionary of Symbols*. New York: Philosophical Library, 1962.

COHN, NORMAN. *The Pursuit of the Millenium*. New Haven, Conn.: Yale Univ. Press, 1973.

CROWLEY, ALEISTER. *The Confessions of Aleister Crowley*. New York: Hill and Wang, Inc., 1970.

CUMONT, FRANZ. *Astrology and Religion Among the Greeks and Romans.* New York: Dover Publishers, 1960.

DE GIVRY, EMILE. *Pictorial Anthology of Witchcraft, Magic and Alchemy.* New Hyde Park, N.Y.: University Books, 1958.

EBON, MARTIN, ed. *The Psychic Reader.* New York: World Publishers, 1969.

ELIADE, MIRCEA. *Myths, Dreams and Mysteries.* New York: Harper and Row, 1967.

ELLIS, ALBERT. *How to Live with a Neurotic.* New York: Crown Publishers, 1975.

———, and HARPER, ROBERT A. *Guide to Rational Living.* Englewood Cliffs, N.J.: Prentice-Hall, Inc., 1961.

*Encyclopedia of Magic and Superstition* (one volume). London: Octopus Books, Ltd., 1974.

*Encyclopedia of Occult Sciences* (one volume). New York: Tudor Publishing Co., 1968.

"The Exorcism Frenzy," *Newsweek* magazine. February 11, 1974.

EYSENCK, H. J. *Sense and Nonsense in Psychology.* Baltimore, Md.: Pelican Books, 1957.

FELDMAN, ARTHUR M., ET AL. *Magic and Superstition in the Jewish Tradition.* Catalogue. Chicago, Ill.: Spertus College of Judaica Press, 1975.

FRAZER, JAMES GEORGE. *The Golden Bough.* New York: Macmillan Co., 1963.

FREUD, SIGMUND. *The Basic Writings of Sigmund Freud.* New York: Modern Library, 1938.

FROMM, ERICH. *Escape from Freedom.* New York: Holt, Rinehart & Winston, Inc., 1941.

GARRETT, EILEEN J. *Sense and Nonsense of Prophecy.* New York: Berkeley Medallion Books, 1968.

GREELEY, ANDREW. *Ecstasy: A Way of Knowing.* Englewood Cliffs, N.J.: Prentice-Hall, Inc., 1974.

GREENE, DANIEL ST. ALBIN. "Satan Lives!" *National Observer.* September 1, 1973.

HAPPOLD, F. C. *Mysticism.* Harmondsworth, Middlesex, England: Penguin Books Ltd., 1963.

HEENAN, EDWARD F., ed. *Mystery, Magic and Miracle.* Englewood Cliffs, N.J.: Prentice-Hall, Inc., 1973.

HILL, DOUGLAS. *Magic and Superstition.* London: Paul Hamlyn, Ltd., 1968.

HUGHES, PENNETHORNE. *Witchcraft.* Harmondsworth, Middlesex, England: Penguin Books Ltd., 1965.

JAMES, WILLIAM. *The Varieties of Religious Experience*. New York: New American Library, Inc., 1958.

JUNG, CARL GUSTAV, ed. *Man and His Symbols*. Garden City, N.Y.: Doubleday & Co., 1964.

KINKEAD, EUGENE. "Is There Another Life After Death?" *Look* magazine. October 20, 1970.

KLEMESRUD, JUDY. "Witchcraft." New York *Times*. October 31, 1969.

LA VEY, ANTON S. *The Satanic Bible*. New York: Avon Books, 1969.

LE SHAN, LAWRENCE. *The Medium, The Mystic and the Physicist*. New York: Viking Press, 1974.

LEWIS, C. S. *The Screwtape Letters*. New York: Macmillan Co., 1961.

LYONS, ARTHUR. *The Second Coming: Satanism in America*. New York: Dodd, Mead & Co., 1970.

MADDOCK, MELVIN. "The New Cults of Madness." *Time* magazine. March 13, 1972.

MASTERS, R. E. L. *Eros and Evil*. New York: Lancer Books, 1969.

MICHELET, JULES. *Satanism and Witchcraft*. New York: Citadel Press, 1939.

MURPHY, GARDNER, ed. *An Outline of Abnormal Psychology*. New York: Modern Library, 1929.

MURRAY, MARGARET A. *The Witch-Cult in Western Europe*. London: Oxford Univ. Press, 1921, 1962.

"The New Cults: A Critique." *The Humanist*. September–October, 1974.

"The Occult Revival." *Time* magazine. June 19, 1972.

OSTRANDER, SHEILA, AND SCHROEDER, LYNN. *Psychic Discoveries Behind the Iron Curtain*. Engelwood Cliffs, N.J.: Prentice-Hall, Inc., 1970.

OURSLER, WILL, AND BANERJEE, H. N. *Lives Unlimited*. Garden City, N.Y.: Doubleday & Co. 1974.

RACHLEFF, OWEN S. *The Occult Conceit*. Chicago, Ill.: H. Regnery & Co., 1971.

———. *Sky Diamonds: The New Astrology*. New York: Hawthorn Books, 1973.

REIK, THEODOR. *Pagan Rites in Judaism*. New York: Crown Publishers, 1964.

RHINE, J. B. *The Reach of the Mind*. New York: William Sloane, 1947.

RHINE, LOUISA. *ESP in Life and Lab*. New York: Macmillan & Co., 1967.

ROBBINS, ROSSELL H. *The Encyclopedia of Witchcraft and Demonology*. New York: Crown Publishers, 1959.

ROSZAK, THEODORE. *Unfinished Animal*. New York: Harper & Row, publishers, 1975.

SANDERS, ED. "Charlie and the Devil." *Esquire* magazine. November 1973.

SENDY, JEAN. *The Coming of the Gods*. New York: Berkeley Publishers, 1970.

"SMITH, ADAM". *Powers of Mind.* New York: Random House, 1975.

SPRAGGETT, ALLEN, and RAUSCHER, WILLIAM V. *Arthur Ford: The Man Who Talked with the Dead.* New York: New American Library, Inc., 1973.

THALHEIMER, ROSS. *Reflections.* New York: Philosophical Library, 1972.

VAN OVER, RAYMOND, ed. *Psychology and Extrasensory Perception.* New York: New American Library, Inc., 1972.

VETTER, GEORGE B. *Magic and Religion.* New York: Philosophical Library, 1973.

WILSON, COLIN. *The Occult.* New York: Random House, 1971.

WYSCHOGROD, EDITH, ed. *The Phenomenon of Death.* New York: Harper & Row, 1973.

ZARETSKY, IRVING I., and LEONE, MARK P. *Religious Movements in Contemporary America.* Princeton, N.J.: Princeton Univ. Press, 1974.